Cancer-Free

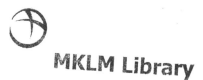

Cancer-Free
30 Who Triumphed Over Cancer Naturally

Compiled and Edited
by the East West Foundation
with Ann Fawcett
and Cynthia Smith

Foreword by Alex Jack

Japan Publications, Inc.
Tokyo • New York

To the memory of Jean and Tony,
who helped start the cancer and diet revolution

Cancer-Free
30 Who Triumphed Over Cancer Naturally
© 1991 by the East West Foundation (cases 4-28) unless otherwise noted
and by Ann Fawcett (cases 1-3).

Note to the reader: Those with health problems are advised to seek the
guidance of a qualified medical or psychological professional in addition
to qualified macrobiotic teacher before implementing any of the dietary or
other approaches presented in this book. It is essential that any reader who
has any reason to suspect serious illness seek appropriate medical, nutritional, or psychological advice promptly. Neither this nor any other related
book should be used as a substitute for qualified care or treatment.

Published by Japan Publications, Inc., Tokyo & New York

Distributors:
UNITED STATES: Kodansha America, Inc., through Farrar, Straus & Gi-
roux, 19 Union Square West, New York, N.Y. 10003. CANADA: Fitzhen-
ry & Whiteside Ltd., 195 Allstate Parkway, Markham, Ontario, L3R 4T8.
BRITISH ISLES AND EUROPEAN CONTINENT: Premier Book Mar-
keting Ltd., 1 Gower Street, London WC1E6HA. AUSTRALIA AND
NEW ZEALAND: Bookwise International, 54 Crittenden Road, Findon,
South Australia 5023. THE FAR EAST AND JAPAN: Japan Publications
Trading Co., Ltd., 1-2-1, Sarugaku-cho, Chiyoda-ku, Tokyo 101.

First Edition: November, 1991
LCCC: 81-060393
ISBN: 0-87040-794-5
Printed in the United States of America

Contents

Part III Medical Research

Part IV Appendixes

Foreword

Since the early 1980s, the relationship between diet and cancer has received increasing scientific investigation and acceptance. In 1982, the National Academy of Sciences, after weighing the evidence, released a 400-page report linking diet with incidence of all of the common cancers (lung, breast, prostate, colon, pancreas, bladder, etc.). They concluded by issuing a set of interim cancer prevention dietary guidelines that recommended increased consumption of whole grains, fruits, and vegetables and decreased consumption of red meat, whole dairy, alcohol, etc. Since then, their recommendations have been adopted by other agencies including the National Cancer Institute and the American Cancer Society.

Meanwhile, Kellogg's and other giant cereal companies have begun to promote fiber, bran, and whole grain products as part of a prudent diet to prevent cancer. When former President Reagan was diagnosed with intestinal polyps (a possible pre-cancerous condition), his physician put him on a special diet that reduced his intake of red meat, white flour, and sugar, and increased his intake of grains, fresh vegetables, and other whole foods.

While the medical and scientific community, as well as segments of the food industry, are now in the forefront of efforts to improve the American diet, much of the impetus to change direction came from educators Michio and Aveline Kushi and from the international macrobiotic community. For nearly four decades, the Kushis and their associates have been promoting whole natural foods as an important measure in the prevention of heart disease, cancer, and other chronic diseases, as well as in the maintenance of personal, family, and social well-being.

In the mid-1970s, when the medical community was more skeptical than it now is about the diet-cancer relationship, the Kushis selected diet and cancer as an important focus for public education. Their educational campaign included:

• Annual conferences on diet and cancer sponsored by the East West Foundation and later the Kushi Foundation.

• Classes on nutrition and chronic disease at the Kushi Institute in Boston and at a network of macrobiotic centers across the country and around the world.

• Articles and case histories in the *East West Journal* and other publications.

• Cooperation with medical research projects such as the Framingham Heart Study, as well as with studies conducted at Harvard Medical School, New England Medical Center, and Tulane School of Public Health and Tropical Medicine.

• Seminars on the principles of macrobiotic health and medicine for physicians, nurses, and other healthcare professionals.

• Meetings at the United Nations, with the World Health Organization, and with government officials in Washington, D.C.

• Publication of books on diet and cancer by major American, European, and international publishers.

Included in this last category are a number of books by ordinary men and women who have recovered from cancer with the apparent assistance of a macrobiotic dietary approach (see bibliography for a complete listing). In many cases, they recount the stories of individuals and their families who would not accept their prognoses as "terminal," or who declined conventional treatments because of their harmful side effects.

Their accounts — dramatic, moving, troubling, inspiring — are like the diaries of our Pilgrim forebears or the pioneers who settled the West. Traversing uncharted territory, often experiencing deep conflicts and divisions within their own households, and confronting skeptical and sometimes hostile powers, they pressed on, made many mistakes, and suffered agonizing personal and professional losses. But in the end, they came to a new awareness of themselves, the origins and causes of their illnesses, and the opportunity of helping others. They transformed their illnesses into health, their ignorance into understanding, and their fear into faith.

The title of this book, *Cancer-Free*, the most recent addition to this library of profiles and personal accounts, refers to this process. Freedom from cancer is not just absence of disease. Freedom from cancer is consciously living in harmony with the environment and the universe as a whole. It is informed by science, deepened by self-reflection, and strengthened through observation and experience of the patterns of nature (encompassed in a unifying principle referred to as "yin and yang"). These patterns of change and balance (see appendix) are so simple that a child can learn them. Yet many of us have lost touch with this simple understanding — as a result of judgment clouded by drugs or alcohol, overly specialized educations, or unthinking dependence on "experts."

The subjects of these chapters, at first, had a hard time grasping that they might have contributed to their own illnesses, or that something as mundane as a change in diet or attitude could make such a profound difference in their outcomes. Yet, like past generations of pioneers, they persevered and came to a deeper appreciation of their difficulties and hardships. In each case, they came to learn from — and even see the positive side — of their illnesses. By taking responsiblity for their own health and destiny, they developed physically, mentally, and spiritually into new people — with greater freedom and awareness and capacity to guide others.

It is also important to understand the limitations of personal accounts such as the ones that follow. They are not part of controlled scientific research studies. For that reason, we have included a brief summary of two scientific studies that were performed to evaluate the effectiveness of macrobiotics. The Tulane study focused on an extremely virulent type of cancer — primary cancer of the pancreas. While the results of that study are inconclusive, it is encouraging to see this type of work being performed. The second study, Dr. Vivien Newbold's, concerned several different advanced malignancies that went into remission following a macrobiotic dietary approach. Though rejected by several medical journals for "insufficient interest" to their readers, it was praised in a recent Congressional Report on alternative cancer therapies which called for further research like

Newbold's to examine the possible therapeutic effects of macrobiotics for cancer patients. (Note: her study includes two new cases of successful recoveries, which combined with the twenty-eight cases presented in Parts I and II, make a total of thirty. There are also duplicates of two cases in Parts I and II and two cases in which the individuals initially recovered, went off macrobiotics and died.)

From a scientific perspective, there are many variables in addition to dietary change that could have affected the outcomes of the cases presented in this book. However, most of these accounts are well documented medically, and it is hoped that, along with the preliminary scientific studies now underway, they will lead to the rigorous randomized clinical dietary intervention trials that will ultimately be needed to conclusively answer the questions of whether proper diet can help to prevent or relieve cancer. This type of research will provide the foundation upon which the medicine of the future will be built, and the articles in this collection are a contribution to that end.

For sharing their personal lives with us, we are grateful to all the persons included in this book and to their families. Ann Fawcett and Cynthia Smith, the writers, are journalists with macrobiotic training, and they are to be commended for their patience and hard work in compiling the first five profiles. Ann and Cynthia visited the subjects and those close to them, often several times and over an extended period of time. A preliminary list of twenty-five questions was prepared for the initial interviews, including the following:

• How did you feel when you were first told that you had cancer?

• How did family members feel and react?

• What was your emotional reaction to your medical treatments?

• How did you learn about macrobiotics?

• What kind of first impressions did you have before you began?

• How did you begin? From a book? By going to a center? Through a friend? A teacher?

• Did you have difficulty with the new way of cooking, in obtaining food supplies, or in getting used to unfamiliar foods?

• What were the reactions of family and friends when you started macrobiotics? What were the comments or reactions of your doctor?

• Did you continue your medical treatments and, if so, for how long?

• When you were medically diagnosed as having no evidence of disease, how did you feel and what were your doctor's comments?

• Besides tumor remission, have you experienced other changes (e.g., intellectual, emotional, in terms of family relations, etc.) in your life as a whole?

• How did your medical expenses compare with those related to your practice of macrobiotics? Did you spend more? Less?

• Have you changed spiritually as a result of your experience?

• What was your diet like before macrobiotics? What foods were you brought up on? As an infant, were you breast-fed or given formula? What kinds of foods did you like or dislike as a child and adult?

• Up to the time of your illness, what were your favorite foods?

• What do you think were the causes of the cancer?

• What do you think caused it to go away?

Originally, the case histories in Part II were to have been included as an appendix to the five longer cases, but as the project developed, it became clear that there were enough for another section. Some of these cases originally appeared in *One Peaceful World*, the newsletter of the One Peaceful World society, and some were specially written for this book. Though not as detailed as the accounts in Part I, they are as powerful and pioneering, and we are grateful for all those who contributed to this section.

Many people contributed to the final shape and outcome of this book. Special thanks are due to Michio and Aveline Kushi for support and encouragement and to Edward Esko, a senior teacher at the Kushi Institute, for overall coordination of this project. Donna Cowan, Carolyn Heidenry, Hisao Kushi, Tom Monte, and Judy Pingryn also contributed to the final macuscript. Lynda Shoup helped with typing, and Gale Jack oversaw the final copyediting and proofreading. Typesetting and production were handled by One Peaceful

World Press in Becket, Mass. with assistance from Dennis Shepard and George Wiel. Finally, we are grateful to Mr. Iwao Yoshizaki and to Mr. Yoshiro Fujiwara, president and vice-president, respectively, of Japan Publications, Inc., the publisher, for their support and encouragement during the completion of this project.

During the last few years, macrobiotics has continued to achieve greater recognition. The *American Medical Association Family Medical Guide* noted: "In general, the macrobiotic diet is a healthful way of eating." Medical research on macrobiotics is continuing at Harvard Medical School, New England Medical Center, University Hospital (in Boston), Tulane School of Public Health and Tropical Medicine, and elsewhere. In the Soviet Union, Michio and Aveline Kushi's books are being translated into Russian, and Soviet medical doctors are beginning to incorporate diet into their treatment of cancer, especially for leukemia, lymphoma, and other malignancies associated with exposure to nuclear radiation. The dietary application of universal principles in East and West may result not only in a cancer-free world but also in a world of greater peace and harmony.

Alex Jack
Becket, Massachusetts
June 1, 1991

Alex Jack is director of One Peaceful World and co-author with Michio Kushi of The Cancer-Prevention Diet. *His most recent book,* Let Food Be Thy Medicine *(One Peaceful World Press, 1991), summarizes 185 scientific and medical studies showing the benefits of macrobiotics for personal and planetary health.*

Part I
Profiles

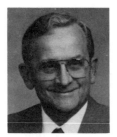

1

Edmund Hanley
Prostate and Bone Cancer

Edmund Hanley, a congenial resident of Muskegon, Michigan, learned he had prostate cancer in January 1980. At the time, he asked his priest to offer a special healing prayer for his recovery. A man of deep abiding faith, Ed has attended 6:30 A.M. mass for over thirty years. Early one morning after mass, in response to Ed's request, the priest led him back into the sacristy of the church where the prayer and accompanying ritual was to be performed. He was hoping for a miracle, an instantaneous healing like the ones attributed to Jesus of Nazareth 2,000 years earlier. Afterwards, however, Ed felt no different. "When I didn't I thought, 'Well, I guess God doesn't have any miracles planned for me.'" Then he laughed and said, "Little did I know."

Two years passed and the cancer began to metastasize very rapidly throughout his body. Doctors designated his cancer at Stage III. He had not undergone an operation or radiation treatments, but was taking the hormone estrogen. At this point Ed decided to try the macrobiotic approach to healing himself. He also decided to stop taking the prescribed hormone pills. One year from the date when he first learned to correctly apply macrobiotic principles to his diet, Ed Hanley was pronounced clear of cancer by medical tests and examination. Though slower in coming than originally expected, Ed believes this was the miracle he asked for, the knowledge of which he gladly shares with others.

Ed was sixty-one and an administrator at Kaydon Corporation, a Muskegon bearing manufacturer, when he learned of the prostate cancer. Married and father of six, his youngest was seventeen at the time. Besides the responsibilities accompanying a large family, he and wife Jeanne had a full social life as well.

Popular as a "stand up comic" (his own description) Ed possesses a repertoire of jokes collected over a lifetime. Consequently he was and still is invited to lend his light-hearted fun to luncheons, conventions, and meetings. Once a member of a barber shop quartet, he also enjoys getting people to sing at parties and other social gatherings. An adept artist with watercolors and woodcarving, in years past he taught classes in watercolors for a Muskegon adult education program. In 1986 he was commissioned by a group of Catholic women to handcarve a wooden statue of St. Francis of Assisi to be presented to their church. An avid cook, after retirement at age sixty-five, Ed took over most of the cooking for Jeanne and himself so Jeanne could continue to sell real estate. In May 1987, when he and Jeanne were interviewed for this story, Ed was sixty-eight. An informed guess places Jeanne to be only a few years younger. At that time both appeared to be in their early fifties. About six months before Ed began eating macrobiotically he became active in a local YMCA athletic and physical fitness program. Today Ed regularly jogs and swims. And though he is officially retired, Ed scoffs when he hears the word in reference to himself. He says, "I'm busier now than I ever was in my life." With a grateful tone in his voice, Ed admits to having the energy of a man in his thirties. Much of this energy is directed towards helping others who have cancer learn to use macrobiotics to heal themselves. Possessing the phenomenal amount of energy he now has was not always the case.

Ed recalls a period when his enthusiasm and energy were at an all-time low. From 1960 to sometime after learning about the prostate cancer, Ed's life followed a pretty weary, hum-drum pattern.

"When I came home at night, I'd pick the paper up, come in the house, lie on the davenport, read the paper and fall asleep. Jeanne would wake me up to tell me it was time for dinner. After dinner we'd put on the T.V. Then I would sit down in the chair, try to finish the paper and go to sleep reading it. Jeanne would wake me at 11:00 and tell me it was time for bed. All the exercise I got was raking the leaves or taking the garbage out."

A major transformation began to take place in Ed when he first learned about his prostate cancer. In 1979 a neighbor told Ed about his own bout with a prostate problem. In fact, Ed was out in the backyard raking leaves at the time when they talked about it. He hadn't seen the man for awhile and asked why. This conversation set a nagging voice going inside Ed's head. It urged him to go to the doctor to have his own prostate checked. "I had gone to my internist a couple of years before and he said my prostate was really enlarged. At that time the doctor explained to me, 'You know, men usually have that problem when they get to be in their sixties.' He suggested I come back at least once a year for a checkup. I hadn't been back in two years." A month later Ed had an appointment with his doctor. "He checked me over and told me, 'There is something hard in your prostate.' He could feel it through the rectum lining with his finger. 'I think you ought to go to a urologist and let him check it out, too.' I had a friend who is a urologist. So a week later I went to an appointment with him. He checked the prostate and said, 'Yeah, there is something hard there, and feels like stones.' He didn't come right out and tell me I had tumors. Neither one of them told me they found tumors. The urologist said, 'I think to be safe we should do a biopsy. I'll make an appointment and see you in the hospital.' The biopsy was performed in another week. A week later the doctor called. 'Ed,' he said, 'I would like to see you this afternoon about three or four o'clock. Can you make it?'

"Sure I can."

"And he added, 'Bring Jeanne along with you.' Then he hung up.

"I thought, 'Wait a minute. Why bring Jeanne with me?' Well, I called Jeanne and she wanted to know 'What's that all about?' Nobody ever says that unless there's something drastically wrong. I couldn't imagine something all that serious."

Remembering her feelings that day Jeanne said, "Sitting in that doctor's office was like going to the guillotine. It was terrible."

Ed said, "The doctor came into the room and he's usually a joker sort of guy. But this time he was all serious and had this folder in his hand. He said, 'Ed, I have got bad news. You have prostate cancer. I think we have good news, too. I think we caught this pretty early. I think we should do a bone scan.'"

When results were back from the bone scan the doctor told him, "Ed, there are hot spots in your skull and pelvis, but I can't tell whether it's cancer. Since we caught it so early, I highly recommend an operation. I will check the lymph nodes in the area. If they are clear we will take the prostate out and then you are all set. The cancer is gone."

"Well, when you know you have cancer it scares the daylights out of you. Anything that the doctor says, that's the way you are going to go. You'll do anything. So I set up to have the operation. On the way home Jeanne said, 'I think we ought to talk to the kids.' They were all over the country . . . in Lansing, Grand Rapids, Haslett, (Michigan) and Denver. They were sympathetic, of course, and were going to keep me in their prayers. Our son Dick, on the other hand, responded differently. Dick has a long time interest in natural healing methods having been a vegetarian for many years." Ed recalls Dick saying, "I think you are crazy."

"I said, 'Thanks a lot, why do you say that?'

"He said, 'You are not going to die tomorrow or probably not next week or maybe not even a year from now. You have all the time in the world to go get a second opinion." Dick also reminded his father that he had complete medical coverage and could do anything he wanted to do. He suggested Ed go to some place like Mayo Clinic or Sloan-Kettering where the latest research on cancer was available. "Jeanne and I talked about that afterwards and Jeanne agreed. She said, 'I think it would be smart to get a second opinion.'" They decided to go to Mayo Clinic. Ed called his internist and told him about this decision. The internist thought that was a good idea, too.

At the Mayo Clinic in Rochester, Minnesota, another bone

scan and other tests were completed. A doctor there then reviewed all the results from bone scans, biopsy slides, blood tests and urinalysis. Ed was surprised when the doctor told him, "No operation for you."

Ed asked, "Why not?"

The doctor replied, "We know you have prostate cancer, but we don't know for sure whether you have bone cancer unless we do a biopsy. And, I'm sure you don't want me to drill a hole in your skull or into your abdomen to get to your pelvis. It's been our experience that with the cancer you have, chances are very good you have bone cancer. When prostate cancer metastisizes it goes into the bone, and removing your prostate would cause it to spread."

"I asked him, 'What am I to do?' He answered, 'If I were in your position, I would just take hormone pills. We don't know how to cure this stuff. We could castrate you and that would slow it down, but the hormone pills will too.' So I said, 'Well, I guess that is what we are going to have to do.' He gave me about ten years of life yet." When Ed returned to Muskegon his internist was also surprised to learn Ed was advised not to have the operation and to only take hormone pills, i.e. estrogen, in the form of diethylstilbestrol. At Ed's request, the internist made a prescription out for the hormone pills, but "he was really miffed," said Ed. "He told me, 'I want you back here in six months and we will do a bone scan and prostate check.' Every time I went in he checked the prostate and then drew a picture of the size he thought the tumors were to have something to refer to the next time. I went there for two years and things were quite dormant. Everything remained the same."

"At the beginning of the third year the cancer began to metastasize. I went in after a bone scan and he told me it was in the lumbar region of my spine. The next time it was in the thoracic area and my ribs. I was still feeling great except when Jeanne and I traveled somewhere in the car. I was so sore down around my pelvis. That must have been the cancer.

"The urologist kept bugging me. He said, 'Ed, I don't know if you realize how serious this is. You have cancer in your prostate. It's metastasized and it's going into your bones.' He kept begging me to get radiation therapy. I kept saying I didn't want the damn stuff. A friend of mine, whom I worked with over at the bearing plant had gone through this. And he was telling me about it. It's just hell. He said he was so darn sick all the time. It was just terrible. He told me, 'If you ever have it, I will come over and hold your hand and at least talk to you.' I thought, 'Lord, I don't need this stuff.' Mainly, I think it was because I felt good. Maybe if I had been in a lot of pain like so many cancer patients, my thoughts would have been different.

"The last time I saw the urologist he said, 'Look, Ed. I made an appointment with you and the radiologist at Hackley Hospital. I want you to go over there and quit horsing around.' I said, 'If it will make you happy, I will do it.'" When Ed got there the radiologist asked Ed, "'What do you want me to do?' I told him, 'I was sent here because you are supposed to give me radiation therapy.' And the doctor replied, 'It's too late for that. You have bone cancer. I can't do you any good.' I couldn't believe what I was hearing. I called the urologists and told him what the radiologist said. Think of all these things that happened to me. The dear Lord was there leading me on. If I had the operation, radiation therapy, all that stuff, think of the horrible situation I would be in today."

"I wasn't afraid to die." Ed explained. "I'm a pretty good Catholic and go to mass everyday. I've seen my family grow up. I've had a good life and happen to think the hereafter is a pretty neat place." One thing that did bother him was leaving Jeanne behind and alone. Strong incentive to really dig in and fight the cancer didn't come, however, until his son David, a psychotherapist, asked to come over and talk with him and Jeanne one evening. During what was an emotional interchange, Ed remembered his son telling him, "Dad, I just feel you are on the way out. I don't see that you are going to live much longer now that the cancer is metastasizing. Here we are getting to be friends and doing things together. I'm just getting to know you and you are going to die." "He broke into tears," Ed said. "We both did. Well, I thought, 'By God, I'm going to fight this thing. I'm not going to let myself die.' He gave me the real desire to get in there and go to work on this even though I didn't have that much faith in macrobiotics at the time.

"When I first found out I had cancer a friend gave me a copy of a *Saturday Evening Post* article about Dr. Sattilaro's recovery from prostate cancer using macrobiotics. (Dr. Sattilaro was chief administrator at Methodist Hospital in Philadelphia at the time.)

"I read that article and wrote to the East West Foundation in Boston for some literature. Material they sent back gave me a rough idea of what a macrobiotic diet consisted of . . . whole grains, fresh vegetables, no meat, no sugar, no white flour, no dairy products or caffeine or alcohol.

"When the third year came and the cancer started to metastasize I kept thinking about macrobiotics. At the Mayo Clinic the doctor said they didn't know how to cure it. Finally I said to Jeanne, 'I've been thinking of giving macrobiotics a try. What do you think about it?' She said, 'I have been thinking about that, too.' That's how we got involved. We started from there." The talk with David gave him that extra push he needed.

July 10, 1983, Ed and Jeanne began macrobiotics on their own by going to a local health food store and getting a couple of books on the subject. One was a cookbook by Wendy Esko. The other was a personal story of a man who healed himself of cancer through macrobiotics. A couple of weeks later the owner of the health food store told them about an anesthetist whose wife had cancer. She was also using macrobiotics in an effort to restore her health after a devastating bout with radiation and chemotherapy. After making contact with them, this doctor and his wife convinced Ed and Jeanne to go to Boston for an interview with a certified macrobiotic teacher and to attend cooking classes. The interview would enable them to know the best foods for Ed's condition and cooking classes would teach Ed and Jeanne the most effective way to prepare them. As many of the foods were prepared from basic unrefined, whole food ingredients and others were entirely new to both of them, cooking classes would be very helpful towards getting Ed and Jeanne off to a strong start. They took the advice, contacted the East West Foundation to set up an appointment and classes, arranged time off from work, packed up their car and drove to Boston.

The Hanleys found their way to the Macrobiotic Learning Center in Brookline, a Boston area town. Lauren Spector, director of the program, took them to meet with senior macrobiotic teacher, Edward Esko, at the East West Foundation. The date was September 12, 1983. Esko explained the relationship between diet and health and outlined the macrobiotic dietary approach, taking into consideration Hanley's constitution and health. From a list of standard macrobiotic foods some foods were emphasized more than others while a few on the list were temporarily restricted. Ed was to eat selected whole grains, fresh vegetables, seaweeds, beans and special soups. He was advised to avoid meat, dairy products, fats, refined sugars, refined flours, caffeine or alcohol.

Ed and Jeanne stayed at the Learning Center for the week they were there taking cooking classes. "During the evenings," Ed said, "ex-cancer patients came and ate with us along with other people. One of these was a registered nurse named Virginia Brown who healed herself of Stage IV melanoma using macrobiotics." Ed talked to her and others like her.*

"I'll tell you, when you meet them in the flesh and hear what bad shape they were in it helps you believe you can recover. It was a good feeling."

Cooking classes at the center were held twice a day for two hours each time. "The week of learning how to cook macrobiotically really helped," said Ed. "It gives you a lot of encouragement. You see the variety of different foods you can come up with even though you are limited to the ingredients you can use. You learn how to cut vegetables a certain way, what to listen and watch for when you are cooking. Lauren took us shopping and showed us the different kinds of cooking utensils, things we would need . . . knives, rice paddles, chopsticks and a salad press. We learned how to make pressed salad by layering vegetables such as cabbage, celery, and carrots with a little salt. They call it pickling and recommend you have it at least twice a week. We bought everything we needed except the pressure cooker (needed to cook brown rice) in Boston. When we prepared to return home, our car was loaded to the brim."

It was September when Ed had the meeting with Mr. Esko. He

---

*Virginia Brown is the author of *Macrobiotic Miracle: How a Vermont Family Overcame Cancer,* with Susan Stayman, Japan Publications, 1984.

wanted to see Ed again in December. When Ed said he couldn't come back East a second time, Esko told him, "There's a doctor outside Chicago. He's a general practitioner and practices macrobiotics. I suggest you see him if you can't come to Boston." Ed called the doctor toward the end of January 1984. They set an appointment for mid-February. The doctor said, "Bring all your bone scans, biopsy slides, films, and any clinical records your urologist has." "My appointment was five months after I had been in Boston and started the diet," Ed recalls. "He looked over all my records including the little drawings of tumors done by the urologist. Then we went into the examination room and he examined my prostate. He said, 'Where are those tumors?' One of the tumors was gone and the other was the size of a pin head. This was a rectal exam, done strictly by feel. He suggested I have ultrasound pictures taken of the prostate by a urologist at University of Chicago Hospital. On March 22, 1984, the doctor took a series of twelve ultrasound pictures and could see no evidence of tumors on my prostate.

"One month later he performed a biopsy of the prostate and found no evidence of cancer cells. A bone scan performed at that time showed a small amount of cancer on my skull and one rib. Then on September 11, 1984, another bone scan was performed and showed no evidence of cancer." It was exactly one year since Ed began the macrobiotic diet suggested to him by Edward Esko in Boston . . . recommendations he strictly followed from that day with the ardent support of his wife Jeanne. After learning Ed was free of cancer Jeanne said, "It felt like Rocky winning." That day in the doctor's office when the news was reported back to him, everyone stopped what they were doing and congratulated them. "The doctor was exhilarated," Ed recalled. "I felt a great weight lift off my shoulders. Then he called me back into the consultation room and said, 'The cancer cells are all gone, but you still have these toxins in your body. If you go back to your old diet, eating your meat, dairy products and these things, it won't be anytime before you'll have the cancer back again. It's going to take a number of years to get rid of these toxins and you will be having discharges from them as your body continues to cleanse itself. Of course, now that the cancer is gone there are things I am going to let you have that you couldn't have before.'" Up to that point Ed could have no oil. He was now allowed to have stir-fry, in which vegetables may be cooked with oil. In November, 1986, the doctor added a few more things to Ed's diet that were not permitted before, such as an occasional imported dark beer, one that is free of chemicals and preservatives.

On the day Ed and Jeanne were told he was clear of cancer, he said, "I don't think we got out of the doctor's office until six o'clock that evening. We got home late. It's a four-hour drive there. The next day we were telling everybody. I told my secretary at work and news rapidly spread through the grapevine. Later I went to the "Y" and told my friends there. So, word got around town in a hurry. People were stopping me all over the place. The phone was ringing off the hook."

Ed Hanley visits the macrobiotic doctor once a year for a checkup. This includes a bone scan, ultrasound scan of the prostate, blood samples and urinalysis. He remains clear of cancer.

Ed and Jeanne's victory did not come without doubts, sacrifice, and radical adjustment in their lives. When Ed began eating macrobiotically, Jeanne did also. Asked "why?," she said, "I didn't think about it. I just knew if he was going to do it, I had to do it with him. There was no question. If he was going to stay on it, he needed the support. It's just like when someone stops smoking and the other one doesn't. I can't imagine doing otherwise. If it was going to be good for him, it was going to be to be good for me. You had to have faith in it." She laughed and added, "I wouldn't want to cook two meals anyway." After they read Wendy Esko's cookbook, *Introducing Macrobiotic Cooking*, and Jean Kohler's book, *Healing Miracles from Macrobiotics*, about Kohler's own recovery from pancreatic cancer, Ed said, "We thought we had enough information to get into this thing."

"We looked up all the things you had to buy," Jeanne recalled. "We bought brown rice, tamari (soy sauce), sunflower seeds as well as other kinds of seeds and sea vegetables . . . all the basic things. I came home, read the cookbook and started with that. Of course nothing tasted like what we were used to. It seemed like a mountain to cross. And I was really afraid if I didn't cook it right, he wasn't going to get the benefit from it. I was really concerned about that. I realize now that it was better than what we were eating whether it was cooked right or not."

At that time food seemed "terribly bland." Ed said, "You even hated sitting down and eating dinner because that's what you were going to eat." He remembers the first meal. "I came home one evening and Jeanne said, 'Wash up and find a place at the table.' So I sat down and she brought this plate in. I don't remember what. It was probably some boiled carrots and boiled rice. And I said, 'What in the world is this?' She replied, 'This is your macrobiotic dinner.' I asked her, 'How in the name of heaven am I going to survive on this for the rest of my life?' So poor Jeanne struggled along for a couple of weeks or longer, trying to prepare things by looking in the cookbook. She kept saying, 'This is terrible. I need some help.' The proprietor of the health food store one day asked Ed, 'What kind of a diet are you on?' And I explained, 'Well, I am trying macrobiotics, but we are having a hard time with it.' Then he told me about an anesthetist and his wife who lived in a little village about fifteen miles from Muskegon. They had gone out to Boston and seen Michio Kushi. When they came home, they brought a macrobiotic cook with them and she taught them how to do the cooking. The proprietor suggested we call them and gave me their name and number." As it turned out, the doctor knew Ed's brother, a Muskegon opthalmologist.

Enthusiastic about macrobiotics, the doctor invited Ed and Jeanne over for dinner and said his wife would teach Jeanne how to do some of the cooking. "So we went and had a really delicious meal. We had fish, brown rice, some vegetables, and some kind of dessert." Jeanne agreed, "It showed me the possiblities of what you can do with the food." The doctor also showed Ed how to toast pumpkin seeds and season them with a little tamari. It was this occasion when the doctor urged Ed and Jeanne to go to Boston to see a macrobiotic counselor and take cooking classes.

When Ed and Jeanne got to Boston, they found they were using too much tamari soy sauce and oil for Ed's condition. Jeanne said, "Up until then I doctored all the food with tamari and had a good stir-fry every night. It was great." Nevertheless, she said, "After we discovered the way it was supposed to taste, it was difficult. At the

Learning Center, the first night we sat down to eat, there were probably about twelve people around the table. There were all these big mounds of food in huge bowls. I wasn't smart. I took huge helpings. It was difficult, especially the sea vegetables, but I figured I'd better eat it because I took all that. Eating this way took time to get used to. Now it's second nature. We are always excited when we find a new recipe to make."

Ed, on the other hand, said, "I like seaweed. The first year I ate a sheet of nori a day." He still eats kombu and wakame pretty regularly in various dishes. Occasionally he makes hijiki, but he is the only one who will eat it because of the stronger flavor. (Each of these is a different type of seaweed). Aside from getting used to the new tastes and flavors, both have enjoyed the different approach to cooking and cutting vegetables. Cooking everything from "scratch" took some effort, though. Jeanne said, "It was funny at first. We had about a hundred pans and a whole bunch of little dishes. We used to laugh about all the pots and pans we used. I don't know why we used all of them. We don't now. We had our rice, beans, greens, and sea vegetables. You have to plan ahead."

Getting the macrobiotic supplies they needed was something of a challenge and also required planning. Some foods were ordered through Mountain Ark, a macrobiotic mail order service in Arkansas, but little by little the local health food store ordered special items and kept them in stock. During the first year on the trips to see the doctor in Illinois, Jeanne and Ed shopped at a health food store there, stocking up whenever they could. Today, they purchase some food items from a store in Grand Rapids. Because more people in the Muskegon area are now involved with macrobiotics, it has become easier and easier to find what they need locally.

Although Jeanne says she didn't mind the newness of macrobiotic practice, Ed said, "It took awhile to remember all the Japanese words for the different foods. That was a little puzzling. When I shopped I wrote them down because if I didn't I'd get to the health food store and couldn't remember what they were. If that happened, what I would do was go over to the book section of the store and get a macrobiotic cookbook off the shelf and look it up. At first it was kind of upsetting."

In addition to getting used to eating a new way, Ed said, "The first month of the diet I felt terrible. So did Jeanne. We both lost weight. In fact I called Edward Esko and told him I felt lousy. He said, 'Just give it time. The weight is going to come back and you are going to feel better.' After about six weeks I did start feeling better and getting my energy back.

"I went down from 168 pounds to 118 pounds in about three months. I was so skinny. I'm 5 feet 7 inches tall. Down at the 'Y' they do skin folds to find out how much fat you have on you. It was so minimal, they could hardly detect any on me. 168 pounds was pretty fat, too. I had a 42" waist. I was probably that heavy from 1960 to 1983." Ed weighs about 135 lbs. today. Jeanne who is 5 feet 1 inch tall went from a size fourteen to a size five during this same period. Like Ed, her weight came back and today she wears size ten and twelve clothing. Neither expected the weight loss. Ed said it scared him to lose it that quickly. Jeanne, on the other hand, said she "loved it." Jeanne said she was not one to be concerned about her weight before or after changing over to macrobiotics. Nevertheless, when she was so thin family and friends were concerned about her health. "So I guess it's better that I put a little weight on," Jeanne added, "They don't worry about me dying, anyhow."

There were some extra benefits Jeanne experienced from the change of diet besides more natural weight balance. She used to have a lot of bladder infections and constipation, ailments she no longer has. Because she has not had to be as strict as Ed, Jeanne admits to "cheating" here and there. She observes when she hasn't eaten right, though, she is subject to hemorrhoids that immediately clear once she returns to eating more macrobiotically.

Ed has also received an unexpected benefit from the macrobiotic dietary program. After the dramatic weight loss in 1984 and 1985, Ed's personal doctor discovered Ed no longer needed or could he safely take, high blood pressure medication first prescribed for him in 1946. When Ed's weight dropped, he began to show extrememely low blood pressure and feel the effects of that. The original doctor who diagnosed Ed's high blood pressure in 1946 died in the intervening years. His new doctor changed the type of medication, but continued to treat Ed for the high blood pressure until these new events occurred. At the time, Ed took three blood pressure pills a day. Under close supervision of his medical doctor, over a three-week period, these were reduced and finally eliminated altogether. Since then Ed's blood pressure remains in a normal range without any medication.

Although the will to survive is essential to overcoming any serious illness, support from others is always a critical factor in a person's recovery. Support came to Ed from several sources.

Throughout his fight to overcome cancer, Ed says the most support came from his wife Jeanne. "From the day we went to Boston and got into macrobiotics, she watched me like a hawk. Even if I looked like I was going to eat something I shouldn't have she'd say, 'Look, it's your life.' But she'd also say, 'I'm here to watch over you. Don't eat that stuff. It isn't good.' And, she tried so hard to cook things that were good and make meals interesting."

Their children also were generally supportive of their father's efforts. When Ed and Jeanne decided to go East to Boston, David and Dick offered to pay their way. David, however, had a period of concern when he saw his parents lose weight so quickly. Dick, on the other hand, realized the weight loss was part of the healing process. He persisted in encouraging his father to stick with it. If any of the other Hanley children had doubts, these were quickly abated when the Chicago-area doctor's examinations began to show good results. Since their Dad's recovery, a couple of them are beginning to incorporate macrobiotic eating principles into their own lives. All of them refer people who have cancer to Ed. When Ed and Jeanne began the diet, however, Jeanne recalls what it was like cooking for them at the time. "I was working full-time and Ed was too. The kids came on the weekends and I cooked two separate meals. They weren't willing to change their eating habits. One Thanksgiving I made a whole turkey dinner. I would do things differently now because I know more and can make it more interesting. And they are more receptive now."

People Ed worked with were also supportive. "They all knew I had cancer. I told them I was going to Boston to a center where they taught macrobiotics. I don't know what they thought, but they seemed willing to do anything to give me a hand. I told my boss we were driving to Boston and I might be gone a week, and he said 'Don't worry about it.' His wife majored in nutrition in college and was quite curious about my diet and what I was eating."

Relatives, on the other hand, posed a different problem altogether. As mentioned earlier, Jeanne's relatives were concerned about the weight loss. In addition, Jeanne said, "They worry about us not getting the right vitamins. We don't eat meat, so to them we are not getting the right food. No matter what you say, they don't understand." Since Ed no longer has cancer, another question also arises, observed Jeanne. "People say, 'Well, now that you don't have cancer anymore why are you staying on the diet?' They don't realize what it is about." It's hard for Jeanne and Ed to get people to understand macrobiotics is a whole way of creating and maintaining health. Macrobiotic principles such as yin and yang are not easy to explain and the diet is different from that of the four basic food groups.

In the face of these obstacles, nevertheless, Jeanne has persisted and even successfully entertained doubtful family members with a macrobiotic menu. On one occasion she served Almond Tofu, a dish where tofu is marinated in soy sauce, peanut butter, ginger, and garlic. This is then added to stir-fried vegetables such as bamboo shoots, celery, pepper, and almonds. It is served on a bed of brown rice. "A lot of them thought it was stroganoff. They ate it." If they didn't like the dish apparently none said so. Knowing her family and reflecting on the event Jeanne said, "We were brave to have them come over and to serve that."

Friends' reactions to the radical change in Ed and Jeanne's diet varied quite a bit. As Ed experienced it, "Our social life went down the tube." When Jeanne and he returned from Boston, Ed said, "Word got around in a hurry that Ed Hanley's on some screwy diet. They don't eat meat anymore or dairy products and cheese. They don't have their martinis and scotch and sodas. These were friends from way back. We used to eat out together and at each others homes. I imagine they felt there wasn't anything we could eat that they would serve. We kind of felt like outcasts. They didn't even bother to ask us."

There were other friends, however, according to Jeanne who

were more understanding. "If we went somewhere, a potluck or something, they would say, 'Bring what you can eat.' And it always ended up that whatever we brought was gone. They all liked it. They knew what we were trying to do and gave us credit for it." In this regard Jeanne said friends were more understanding than family. "We picked friends to come over and try our meals. Some were great and really appreciated it, but never actually went on the diet. We were trying to prove to them there was food you could eat that didn't have to be meat."

Friends in their church group were especially encouraging. A group of people attending 6:30 A.M. mass often have breakfast together, particularly on Friday mornings. They regularly meet at the same restaurant. Ed and Jeanne bring kukicha, a non-caffeine Japanese twig tea, in a tea bag. There they ask for a pot of hot water for it. In this way Jeanne and Ed are still able to join these friends.

Ed commented,"They were never ones to knock the diet." Church group friends always let him and Jeanne know they were welcome, asked about his progress, and were glad to hear what it was. Also important, Ed said, "When there was anything they thought we could share or fun things to do, they were always there to include us in it. They never let us down. They accepted us 100 percent. If the diet seemed strange to them, they never said so."

Because Ed's brother is an eye doctor, one component of his social circle includes quite a few Muskegon medical doctors of various specialties. Ed is close to his brother and describes him as being "a neat guy." Ed's choice to take up macrobiotics proved awkward for both of them. "The doctors in town found it real difficult to believe I was going to recover. When confronted with a full account of Ed's medical history, i.e. biopsies, bone scans, etc. Ed says, "There are some people (including doctors) who cannot accept the fact I recovered from cancer." This skepticism, however, proved to be one of several strong motivating influences enabling Ed to stick so tightly to macrobiotic dietary guidelines that first critical year. "Whenever I went to Illinois for a checkup, people would ask Jeanne, 'How's he coming along? What condition is he in?' It was kind of nerve racking because I wanted so much to prove to them it works, especially with all those doctors watching us. It kept me going." Today

Ed still has occasion to meet the doctors who initially provided his diagnosis and medical care prior to starting macrobiotics. Generally, he avoids the subject of his cancer recovery. He cites, for example, "If we are at my brother's party and doctors are there, we don't talk about my condition. It's like talking politics, Republican or Democrat. You know how loud you can get. You lose more friends that way."

In spite of this, his commitment to assist anyone who comes to him for information about macrobiotics has attracted local publicity. In July 1985 the *Muskegon Chronicle* ran a front page story on Ed's recovery in a Sunday edition. Four days later, the *Chronicle* printed a Muskegon doctor's rebuttal in the "My Turn" column. About four weeks after that the Illinois doctor responded to both articles, providing further explanation about macrobiotics and emphasizing that in his practice, he used "a broad range of tools — all the convenient medical tools and techniques, as well as a very profound concern for diet, stress management, physical conditioning, etc."

A month after the doctor expressed his views and concerns in the "My Turn" column, Ed told his own story in the sincere, straightforward manner that is his style. The publicity in the Muskegon newspaper, however, left him cautious. In spite of this he remains willing to help in any way he can if someone asks him about macrobiotics and cancer. It's also encouraging to him to know personally one young physician who, through acquaintance with Ed, decided to return to school to study nutrition and its role in creating health. In addition, regarding the validity of macrobiotics, the urologist at the University of Chicago told Ed, "You have made a believer of me." At the conclusion of the ultrasound and biopsy tests conducted on Ed's prostate, the doctor carefully questioned Ed about treatment history of the tumors. It was the urologist's tests that first showed conclusively Ed was free of cancer. Ed told the doctor he had not undergone the usual operation or radiation treatment. Also, he had discontinued taking three daily tablets of the hormone treatment several months earlier. In the *Muskegon Chronicle* "My Turn" column Ed wrote, "It was the urologist's opinion that over this long period of time without them, the pills could not be given credit" for his recovery from cancer. The doctor had previously run similar tests on other patients relieved of cancer who, like Ed, followed macrobiotic diets. Unlike him, however, the others had operations, chemotherapy, radiation and/or hormone pills depending on the type of cancer. Confronted with these facts, the role of the macrobiotic dietary program in the reduction of Ed's prostate tumors was evident to the urologist.

Important as eating macrobiotically was to Ed's recovery though, he is first to tell you prayer and faith is the foundation upon which all his efforts to defeat cancer rested. "If you have faith, the Holy Spirit is going to help you. I feel God is with me." And he also believes the prayers of others helped, too. "There is a time during the 6:30 A.M. mass when the priest asks if anyone has anything they would like to ask others to pray for. If you have any problems, we usually offer up whatever problems we have. We ask everybody else in the community to pray for us and we pray for them, too." For Ed, going to mass and taking communion is an important part of his prayer life. "If I don't go to mass during the morning every day, I just don't feel like I have all my clothes on. I don't feel like the day started right." He also adds, "All through my experience, knowing I had cancer and getting rid of it, I just felt the Lord led me because of the fact I never had operations, chemo, or radiation." Coping with the knowledge he had cancer was a tough challenge. "When I was at work it seemed like voices were constantly telling me 'You've got cancer; you've got cancer; you've got cancer.'"

Intertwined with prayer, he made a conscious effort to cultivate a positive mental attitude. Norman Cousins' book *Anatomy Of An Illness* proved particularly helpful to Ed for this purpose. Cousins wrote about how he himself overcame a terminal illness with laughter. In it he said, "Healing is strongest when the mind is most positive." Ed also discovered if he kept busy doing what he loved to do he felt better. "God gave me the talent to do art work and to work with tools. So I found whenever I would sit down and do a watercolor or teach a class in watercolor, any problems just disappeared. Giving to others through sharing personal talents lightens the weight of the worry, too," he observed.

At the time newspaper articles also emphasized the role of exercise in reducing stress. With encouragement from his son John, who lives in Denver, Ed became involved in exercise programs at the local YMCA. For Ed's birthday in March 1983 a few months before Ed started macrobiotics, John gave Ed a years's membership at the "Y". The gift turned out to be a spectacular success due to Hanley's own enthusiastic participation. He started out with a daily after work "Happy Hour" exercise group designed for business people like himself. From there Ed branched out to swimming and "every other class you can imagine." When he went to Boston, Ed Esko wanted to know what kinds of things Ed was doing to take care of himself. Ed told him about going to the "Y". "He thought it was great and suggested I continue." This activity would complement the recommended macrobiotic dietary program. As time went on Ed became so proficient, he was asked to be an instructor at the "Y". One of the many amusing stories Ed tells is about an exercise class he taught when he was sixty-three, shortly after he learned he was free of cancer. "There was a bunch of college kids that came to the 'Y' and they got credit for gym by taking this class I was teaching. We warmed up, stretched, exercised, and jogged for twenty minutes. One night, at the beginning of a new class, the college students were warming up when a man came in who didn't know I was the instructor. He looked at me as we were jogging around and said, 'Well, at least there is somebody here I can keep up with.' And a young guy running by me knew who I was and said, 'I wouldn't count on that buddy.' The man found out later that I was teaching the class." Ed laughed as he remembered that day. "He was an old guy like me, and here were all these kids." Since then Ed has taught many different kinds of classes including classes conducted in the pool for people with arthritis and hip replacements. "I had an hour of various water exercises. In the water you are buoyed up. Jogging in the pool you don't get the pounding you do when you are not in water. Then I started another class in the pool for people who wanted aerobics. With water working against you, you are really working hard." Ed continues to exercise regularly because he knows how important it is for maintaining a healthy balance in his life.

Ed loved the kind of food he grew up on. "My mother was a good German cook, serving lots of meat, lots of cabbage, potatoes, and gravies. But they were really greasy." Jeanne's mother was German and she, too, cooked similar food although Jeanne recalls roast beef and Yorkshire pudding as well as the gravies. Both admit to missing the foods they were raised on and continued to eat as adults. Today, however, Ed says, "What I discovered through reading is that I brought on my own cancer from all the meat and dairy products. I loved cheese, too. Every day I used to eat at least one meal that had cheese. I was eating meat at every meal. In the morning I had bacon or sausage and eggs. I didn't like oatmeal. I would have a dish of cereal with milk on it. I used to drink a lot of milk. At lunch time I would have a hamburger, lunch meat, or leftover roast. Then in the evening it was more meat, steak, roast, ham, or whatever. My favorite food was Coney Island hot dogs. There is a place in town where they make really delicious hot dogs and put chili on them with lots of onions. The chili had lots of hamburger in it. But I also loved pot roast, mashed potatoes, gravy and any vegetable. My mother used to take pork chops and cook them in sauerkraut. We would have mashed potatoes with lots of butter on them; you can get an idea of the kind of food I liked. And, of course, there were desserts like apple pie with some real strong cheese." During the depression years his mother also prepared a lot of casseroles made with spaghetti or macaroni. The traditional German dark breads such as pumpernickel and rye were replaced with white bread. There were, however, other traditional dishes that remained unchanged. "She was pretty proud of all her recipes and the cooking she did. Apparently, those were handed down and brought over from the old country." One dish they had frequently didn't come over, Ed remembers. "Mother used to make something like Boston baked beans, with lots of brown sugar and a real thick fatty bacon. She also made a very good vegetable soup. If we had chicken or turkey, she used the carcass to make soup. There was a lot of noodle soup. We never went hungry. The things she had filled you up for the time being. There was always some dessert. You know kids. They will hurry up and eat the rest of their meal so they can eat dessert." Today Ed is very conscious of the importance of chewing his food well as an aid to digestion. When he started practicing macrobiotics he became aware of how fast he finished a meal. Recalling childhood desserts he said, "Maybe that was why I became such a fast eater. Today he eats with chopsticks and feels this helps him to eat more slowly and chew food thoroughly.

Ed no longer eats desserts sweetened with white sugar or corn syrup. Even still, occasionally he and Jeanne make treats for themselves with barley malt, rice syrup, and apple juice . . . including apple pie. "I try different crusts made with whole wheat flour. It's not like Mother used to make . . . made with all that lard and nice and flaky. Nevertheless, it's suitable. I like it." His pie filling has undergone various trial and error changes too. With apples he adds chopped dried apricots and raisins. The apricots and raisins are soaked first before he cuts them up. "If I have an eight-inch pie tin, I take a cup of apple juice and add about a quarter cup of barley malt or rice syrup. The barley malt gives more flavor. I mix those together on the stove, heat them and add a couple of heaping teaspoons of arrowroot (a thickener similar to corn starch). First though, I put the arrowroot in a little saucer and dilute it with some apple juice. Then I gradually add it to the pan of apple juice and sweetener till it's almost thickened like a pudding. After that I pour it in with the fruits, stir it all around and put that into the pie shell. I take some sunflower seeds and sprinkle them over everything and put the top crust on the pie. This goes into the oven for fifty minutes." An enthusiastic cook, it's apparent when Ed shares his recipes that eating the results is as much pleasure as the preparation and cooking. He enjoys the challenge of learning how to take the unfamiliar ingredients and turn them into a delicious creation. Jeanne and he both seem to enjoy the adventure and discovery of all the new dishes they have developed or tested.

Before Ed started macrobiotics he took vitamins acquired from the friend who brought him the article about Dr. Sattilaro. He stopped taking them once he began the special macrobiotic dietary program Esko outlined for him. Ed feels confident he is getting the vitamins he needs from the food he eats and no longer needs them. Blood tests taken during checkups with his doctor confirmed this.

Prior to starting macrobiotics, Ed underwent a series of colonics. "It was about six months after learning I had cancer. My daughter was having some problems and went to a nurse for a colonic. She told the nurse about my cancer. The nurse suggested to Barb I ought to come and have colonics. I asked Barb, 'What is a colonic?' She said, 'It's a high powered enema.' 'I'm not going to do that.' Finally, Barb said, 'Look, there are all kinds of guys who go to this nurse.' She talked me into it. I bet I had twenty of them. The nurse would tell me about all the things she was getting out of my colon. There's a tube where all this waste matter is taken out and a section of glass where she could see these things passing by. She said, 'Ed, can you get up here and look over?' You lie on your side while it's being done. So I looked over. Going through the tube at the bottom was a sediment, like sand at Lake Michigan. I said, 'What the heck is that?' I forgot exactly what she told me, but one of my organs was discharging that stuff. It really cleaned me out. I didn't feel it hurt me.

"If you eat all the meat I ate, the thing we learn is a lot of that putrifies in your colon. It just stays there and become toxic. The colon is where all the nourishment is taken out of the food, absorbed into your bloodstream and carried around to all the cells of your body. So this colonic treatment got rid of a lot of the toxins in my colon. I feel now if I had been on the macrobiotic diet, I wouldn't have needed colonics. You can't believe it. When I first got into macrobiotics, I was having bowel movements four times a day. I thought, 'Good grief! I can't have all this food in me. I couldn't have eaten all that,' but I did. You don't have any trouble with bowel movements eating this way."

Looking at the economics of macrobiotics was a revelation for Ed. Before he began macrobiotics, Ed figured the doctor's fees plus going to Mayo Clinic, bone scans, and prostate exams cost about $8,000. When he considered this he thought. "Gee, is that all?" Later he said, "When you stop and think about all the people with cancer who have an operation or radiation, they are in the hospital for about two days and the $8,000 is already down the tubes." Both Ed and Jeanne have also seen a decrease in food bills. Jeanne said, "Even though we are eating fresh vegetables and buying health food I know our food budget has been cut in half. I was also spending $2 a day on soft drinks and more for snack foods. Then there was meat and prepared foods. I was working and would come home and take something out of a box." Like others, Jeanne and Ed find meals prepared from basic, whole food ingredients cost less. At the same time these foods also offer more health sustaining nutrition for the food dollar spent than highly refined, prepackaged "convenience" foods.

Ed says he spends a lot of time cooking or talking about food. Typically for breakfast he prepares brown rice in a pressure cooker. He often adds chickpeas and kombu (a sea vegetable). A miso-lentil-vegetable soup accompanies it with a pot of hot Japanese twig tea. Over breakfast he talked about changes in his life and himself since he learned he had cancer and started macrobiotics. Energetic and sociable though Ed obviously is, it's apparent his life has a solid foundation.

There is a quiet peacefulness about both Ed and Jeanne Hanley, a presence that pervades their comfortable home, their kitchen and the food coming from it. Ed readily admits he was not always this way. "I used to have a hot temper, but now I can keep my cool. I used to get so upset I would tremble. I don't have that problem anymore." Ed says that he blew up over things his kids did, at work and on other occasions. And though he says things still bother him every now and then, he handles it differently. "I stop and think about it. One thing I think is, life is short and I haven't got that much time left. Why should I make it unpleasant by being angry with other people and making them feel bad? Just make it a happy world; that's my attitude now. I think the diet and eating like I have has a lot to do with that. Before, I was always tired, no energy. I would fly off the handle. Now I enjoy the kids. We are around them much more. I think they feel it, too. About his relationship with Jeanne, Ed said, "There were things I did that apparently antagonized her, but I don't seem to be doing them anymore. At least I hope I am not doing them. We are real compatible. We enjoy life together. We share things. We travel together." In fact, they have been sharing household tasks since Jeanne started working in her father's real estate office twenty years ago, when their youngest was five. Though Jeanne did the bulk of cooking prior to their beginning macrobiotics, back then Ed said, "Whoever came home first would start the dinner. If washing had to be done and you were downstairs by the washing machine, you threw it in. If it needed to be dried, you'd dry it." This practice continues today. "I'll iron her things and she will iron mine and so forth,' added Ed. "I have so much energy, too. I get up early, but I can go to bed at quarter after eleven and not be tired. The really neat thing is I can get into bed, kiss Jeanne good night, say my prayers, turn over and I am asleep. Normally I am awake before the alarm goes off at 5:00 or 5:15." Jeanne has also experienced a definite increase in her level of energy though the number of hours of sleep she needs varied depending on the activities of a given period.

After Ed learned he had cancer one thought constantly with him was, "What should I do to make good use of my time?" As a consequence of that reflection Ed says, "I just can't stand to waste time." But his priorities for how to use that time didn't really shift until he was free of cancer. In the July 7, 1985, *Muskegon Chronicle* article Ed remarked, "The dear Lord had his hand on my shoulder during all this. I believe he saved me for some reason. And, it wasn't to just sit around on my doop-ah like so many other retirees." During the May 1987 interview for this story he referred again to the pact he made with God. "I said if I should recover, I would certainly help anyone who asked me to help them." As a result of this vow, Ed was drawn into the many activities that still occupy him today. He is frequently asked to give talks about his cancer recovery and macrobiotics. He averages one or two a month.

The first request was a turning point that helped him realize he could once again join others at group luncheons. "I had been teaching physical fitness at the 'Y' and John Usmial, the fellow in charge of the fitness program, asked me if I would come talk to a service club to which he belonged. I said, 'Well, you know I probably can't eat your food, but is it all right if I bring my own?'

"He replied, 'I guess so. I don't know why not.' So I made a sushi roll with the brown rice, seaweed and vegetables. Then I brought an apple, rice cake and tea bag (made with Japanese twig tea). They had us seated at round tables with five or six at a table. First came the salad. After I ate the salad, the catering service people began bringing in a plate of food for each person. There was some kind of meat with vegetables, gravy and mashed potatoes. Finally I said, 'Can I just have a clean plate with nothing on it?' In disbelief the lady asked, 'A clean plate with nothing on it?' All these guys looked at me like, 'What's the matter with this character?' So she brought in a plate and laid it down. I had my brown bag on the floor next to my chair and I picked it up, took out the sushi roll, then the apple and the rice cake. All these guys looked at this. Then one of them looked at me. He said, 'What the hell is that?'" Seeing the humor in the situation Ed laughed as he recalled that afternoon. "I explained what it was. 'It's a sushi roll.' Then I sliced a little wheel off the roll and asked if they would like to try it. I passed one around and each one took a little out of that and we had a terrific discussion about macrobiotics. After we ate, I had a lot of attention from the audience during the talk, too. That convinced me. There was no reason I couldn't go out to public dinners. I could have fish, salad and a vegetable. If there was anything else served, then I'd just ignore it, or hand it to the guy next to me. We have our kukicha tea bag and it isn't that bad. You get them in health food stores. With one of these bags you can make a quart of tea." Ed asks for the usual hot water in a little tea pot and he's set. If Jeanne is with him one tea bag serves the two of them easily.

"I was giving a talk at a Rotary Club not long ago and this fellow had a question. I said 'What's that?' He responded, 'Here we are eating this steak. (I was eating fish.) How do you feel about that?' 'Well,' I replied, 'to tell you the truth, I was sitting here thinking, 'You poor guy. You are killing yourself.' And they all laughed. I was sincere. That's really the way I feel looking at them eating all that ice cream, cake and desserts. I think, 'You poor souls, you don't know what you are doing.'"

As word got around Muskegon about Ed's remarkable recovery, Ed said, "People would stop and question me about it or call me on the phone. Finally it got to where I was invited to come and give more talks." He also finds himself spending a lot of time with individuals on the phone or in person. "My policy is if someone wants to learn about macrobiotics I'm delighted to talk about it. I will not go to someone I hear about who has cancer and say, 'You ought to get into macrobiotics.' You know, you can lead a horse to water, but you can't make it drink. I have so many asking for my help that I don't have to go out soliciting for any."

In response to this interest and need, Ed and Jeanne started a support group in their home. "There was a fellow who had cancer and wanted to get into macrobiotics, so I set him up. He went to see a counselor at the East West Foundation and took cooking classes at the Learning Center. There were others, too. When I had cancer we had no support at all. We thought there was no one around here that could help us. When we did find someone it made such a difference. That's why we started this support group. When we started we had about half a dozen people. Every month that half dozen would bring someone else until we got such a large group I suggested we find a hall. One couple said, 'We belong to a Methodist church over in North Muskegon and I know we can use their facility.' So we went there and have been going there once a month ever since. It's a potluck dinner.

"When the articles came out in the newspapers about me, they were published in Grand Rapids, too. People started a support group there as a result. They must have the equivalent in membership as we do here. Of the people who come most have cancer. Of course, there are others who are just interested in being healthy. They know they shouldn't be eating some of the things they do. But if not that, what can you eat? You tell them they can have whole grains, vegetables, seaweeds, nuts and seeds, and then they want to know how to prepare anything like that. It's really amazing when you come to this potluck. It's a pretty well-balanced meal with a great variety of dishes and even desserts. When people find all these delicious things you can have, it changes their whole attitude about it.

"There's also a speaker each month. When we first started I was generally the speaker. People would have all sorts of questions I would handle as best I could. Now, however, I have a speaker come. This month we have a speaker on biofeedback and stress management who works out of one of the local hospitals. After that, next month there will be a homeopathic doctor." In addition to arranging speakers for the group, Ed acts as general coordinator, and keeps track of dues charged to cover newsletter costs. Taking dues also helps him keep track of who comes regularly.

Aside from the support group, many individuals ask for his help. "For some people I have gone over to their homes, talked to them and even showed them how to prepare the foods. I give them a list of foods they need to start and some recipes." Responding to numerous requests, Ed and Jeanne have also conducted two or three cooking classes in their home and one at the "Y."

He does this, he said, because "When I left my session with Esko, I knew what foods I could have, how much and when, but not how to cook them. If it hadn't been for the Learning Center we would be like everybody else. If people just go to a counselor, without attending a seminar or cooking class, they don't know how to cook the food. They come back here and before you know it they are helpless. They need help and that's where the support group comes in. So many of us are able to help them." Ed says he gets a call nearly everyday from someone in Muskegon wanting help. "I tell them, 'I will do all I can for you.' but I recommend you see a macrobiotic teacher who is qualified by the Kushi Institute."

There are several points of frustration Ed experiences by making himself so open to others. One in particular is, "They want to know what this 'diet' is. I tell them, 'Look it isn't a diet. It depends on the condition you are in. If you have a degenerative disease the diet depends on what kind of disease you have.' I tell them, basically the food all of us eat is similar. However, there may be some things one person can have and another shouldn't have for a while. I also tell them I'm not a counselor, and am not qualified to tell you what you should or shouldn't have."

Perhaps Ed's biggest frustration comes from people, especially his friends, who have gone to a counselor, received an appropriate macrobiotic diet for their condition and then don't stick to it 100 percent, as is necessary in such extreme conditions as cancer. It also bothers Ed when he learns about a friend with prostate cancer who knows about Ed's own recovery, but doesn't consider macrobiotics. "People just don't want to give up their little goodies, like drinks, steaks and all that stuff. That means more to them than getting healthy."

Calls to Ed are not limited to those in Muskegon. "While we were in Boston, Lauren Specter asked, 'Can we give out your name and phone number to other people who would like to talk to someone who is practicing macrobiotics?' I said, 'Sure.' Same with the health food store fellow and my kids. I get calls from all over the

United States and Canada. I have had calls from California, Canada, Maine, and way down in Florida. I use the International Macrobiotic Directory to help them find the nearest center. I even had a woman over in Austria who wrote me a letter and wanted to know. Some relative sent her this article about me, and, by golly, there was an address for a center in the directory that I could give her in Austria!"

Besides this Ed says, "I pray for them. They tell you to keep them in your prayers and so I do that. I get calls usually from a member of the family. They call and tell me about a relative with cancer and in the hospital. If requested, I will go to the hospital, talk with them and take a book with me, usually Dr. Sattilaro's *Recalled By Life*. I've got several copies around town and lose track of them. People pass them around. There's often somebody else who wants to read it."

Ed plans to continue with these activities and in the future he wants to write his own book about his experience. The book will also outline guidelines on how to form a macrobiotic support group. In addition, he wants to produce his own cookbook plus figure out a menu for everyday of the week in preparation for conducting more cooking classes.

Considering all Ed has laid out for himself to do, he has come a long way from the days when he only had energy to fall asleep on the living room couch. The miracle healing he asked for and received continues to spread outward like ripples caused by one smooth pebble thrown into a quiet pond.

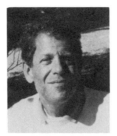

2

Michael Shanik
Malignant Melanoma

In mid-February 1985, Michael Shanik, a successful Florida businessman, learned he had malignant melanoma. In his early forties at the time, he was given three to six months to live. Michael was stunned by the news. Mickey McKay, Michael's wife, was a runner and held a longtime interest in nutrition and health. Some months earlier an architect friend told Mickey about macrobiotics. Together Michael and she considered the options facing him and decided to give this whole food-focused diet a try. The decision saved Michael's life. After strictly eating macrobiotics for four months, in June, Michael appeared to be well into recovery. Continuing to apply macrobiotics principles to his diet, Michael was found free of disease by medical examination and blood tests in September 1985. Medical tests and examinations performed every six months continue to show he no longer has cancer. Michael maintains a file of letters from doctors with xerox copies of lab reports documenting his original diagnosis and incredible recovery. When interviewed for this article in September 1987, his latest blood work at that time was done in May 1987. As reported in a letter to Michael from his examining physician, "A complete twenty-seven channel chemical profile,

CBC with differential urinalysis and CEA were all within normal limits." Survival rate for this type of cancer currently is between 10 percent and 20 percent. It is an aggressive form of cancer and progresses quickly. In spite of these grim facts, at this writing in May 1988, Michael Shanik is alive, healthy and can easily bicycle thirty to fifty miles on a weekend.

In Michael's encounter with cancer, there was no time to hesitate or doubt whether macrobiotics would work for him. His triumph over cancer has been one requiring a thorough commitment to this course of action and teamwork between he and Mickey. The victory belongs to them both. Together they were backed to the edge of an abyss and with firm resolve did not give in to the fear, despair, and panic both felt. Their story is one of single-minded courage.

At the time of diagnosis, both Michael and Mickey were marketing representatives for a design firm in the Miami Gold Cost area. They lived in Boca Raton with Mickey's two children from a previous marriage, Andrea and Christopher. Andrea was in high school and Christopher in junior high. Today, their home is on Siesta Key, part of Sarasota. Three or four steps from a glassed-in family room is a large pond bordered by lush, tropical trees and shrubs native to the area. Thick undergrowth provides total privacy for them, their family and an abundant variety of wild birds who also claim the pond as their permanent or "wintering over" home. One can sit in this family room and be greeted by the stately presence of a Great Blue Heron only several feet away. The outdoors merges with and complements the quiet, gracious elegance of Michael and Mickey's home. Ceiling fans stir the warm, humid, Florida air. In this pleasant environment, Michael and Mickey sat on separate occasions and shared the details of Michael's encounter with cancer.

The year before receiving the cancer diagnosis Michael went to a general surgeon to have a belt-line mole removed. "At the same time the doctor did that procedure in his office," Michael recalled, "I mentioned I had a bump behind my ear on my scalp. I asked if he would look at it. He did and wanted to know if it bothered me. I said, "No." He replied, "Well, if it doesn't, leave it alone." So a year passed, and I noticed the bump was getting larger and that it started hurting. It was irritating me. I noticed this because I was involved with skeet and trap shooting at the time and wore ear protectors. These rubbed against the bump and hurt."

"So again, I went to the same surgeon. He looked at it and said, "It is probably a degenerated lymph node. If it's bothering you and it's painful, it should come out. This can be done in day surgery. It's no big deal."

"The day after Valentine's Day," Mickey said, " I took Michael to the hospital in the morning as an out-patient. Neither of us were anticipating anything. I was working in West Palm Beach where the hospital was, so I went and made one or two appointments." When Michael recovered from anesthesia, the doctor confirmed the lump was a degenerative lymph node. Again the doctor assured Michael it wasn't anything serious, but as a matter of routine he was sending it to Pathology for tests. "That was Friday," Michael said. "On Monday, I got a call at the office from the doctor saying he wanted to see both Mickey and me. He suspected malignant melanoma. He wouldn't give me anymore details than that. He didn't have to say anymore. I knew what that meant."

When Michael arrived home, however, Mickey said, "He was nervous because there was something pending. We didn't know exactly what malignant melanoma was. So we went to the library and checked out several books on cancer and a couple on malignant melanoma. We brought them home and immediately opened them up. That's when we became uncomfortable with the whole thing. The survival rate was 5 to 7 percent, never more than this. Most of the books were seven to ten years old. So I thought even though recovery from malignant melanoma looks slim, perhaps the chances for survival have improved since then." Earlier that afternoon Mickey looked at books she had on macrobiotics. One was titled, *Cancer and Heart Disease: The Macrobiotic Approach to Degenerative Disorders* by Michio Kushi and his associates. This included case histories of people who healed themselves of cancer and heart disease using macrobiotic principles applied to their diet and lifestyle. By the end of that evening Mickey said, "I had macrobiotics on the one hand and the library information on the other. It seemed as though macrobiotics would take care of the problem. From the medical information in the library books, however, Michael was a goner. The next day, Tuesday, we went to the doctor's office. On the way there I had Michael look at the book on macrobiotics and consider it as a possibility. At the office, both Michael's doctor and his partner were present. The doctor said it was definitely malignant melanoma. The lab report confirmed it and prognosis was poor."

He also told Michael and Mickey that chemotherapy does not work on this type of cancer; only surgery might help. First, however, they had to locate the primary site. The cells from the degenerated lymph node were secondary site cells. This meant the cancer came from another area. The doctors wanted to reopen the area from which the bump was removed. They indicated, however, the primary site might be undetectable. Given this strong possibility, they said Michael had three to six months to live. "Still , as a precaution, the doctors suggested extensive surgery. To prepare for this, there was a laundry list of things Michael was to do," said Mickey. "He had to see an opthalmologist specializing in eyes, ears, nose, and throat and a dermatologist who would have to go over every inch of his skin." The doctors wanted many more tests conducted in a attempt to locate the primary site. The following day Michael made appointments with these doctors. "At that time," Michael said, "I also selected an oncologist in West Palm Beach and another in Fort Lauderdale. I chose two so I could have two opinions. They agreed the tests should continue and more samples from the removed growth be sent to other labs rather than the one at little Del Ray Beach Hospital. So samples were sent to the University of Pennsylvania, University of Miami and Brower General Hospital. Miami had probably the most sophisticated testing machine for staining and detecting melanoma. They all verified the presence of melanoma. This period of tests went on for a week to ten days."

The same day, after the doctors told Michael he had melanoma, he and Mickey went to a health food store. Mickey recalled, "We were unsure of macrobiotics because we didn't know much about it. One thing we were sure of though was that Michael's chances were slim to none, according to the doctors, where macrobiotics offered us some hope." At the store, they purchased their first whole grains, beans, and other macrobiotic supplies. As Michael remembered,

"The fellow who was helping us was the owner. We explained to him the problem. He said, 'You know, there is a fellow who comes in here often who has the same situation you do and has been living with this for two years.' He wouldn't give us the man's phone number, but took my office number. I headed back to the office after leaving the health food store and the phone rang. It was Alan Jacobs, the man who had malignant melanoma. The fact he had it and was still alive after two years was pretty incredible given the nature of this type of cancer and the statistics. Alan was my inspiration. He was using the macrobiotic approach to heal himself of cancer. If he could do it, I could do it. That was the ray of hope I needed. *The Cancer-Prevention Diet* (by Michio Kushi with Alex Jack) and Virginia Brown's book *Macrobiotic Miracle* also helped." These were books he and Mickey bought at the health food store. Virginia Brown's book was especially significant to Michael.

In 1978, Virginia Brown, a registered nurse, was diagnosed as having malignant melanoma (Stage IV). Physicians at Vermont Medical Center in Burlington told her that without surgery she had only six months to live. Through eating macrobiotically, she was able to recover fully without surgery or other medical intervention. Her story plus the many successful case histories included in *The Cancer-Prevention Diet* gave Michael a positive perspective on the possibility of surviving cancer. This book also gave instructions on how to go about it. Wednesday, the day after learning Michael had cancer, Mickey also called the Macrobiotic Foundation in Miami and made an appointment to see Lino Stanchich, a macrobiotic counselor. The appointment was Thursday of the next week. "I told them about the case, but they didn't have recommendations until we saw Lino. So I took it upon myself. I felt we should begin eating macrobiotically immediately." Looking back, Michael said, "We cooked about a week using the standard macrobiotic diet without real guidelines. In the meantime, I was having all these (medical) tests. They were coming to an end when we saw Lino." During that meeting Lino Stanchich explained how Michael and Mickey could apply macrobiotic principles and helped tailor a diet for Michael's personal needs. He emphasized their need to prepare food on a gas stove.

In macrobiotics, energy properties in food, the body and environment are important factors in creating health as well a disease. Cooking with electric appliances charges the food with chaotic energy and is detrimental to an individual's health. In traditional Western and Oriental medicine, from which macrobiotic teachings draw heavily, the Ki or energy flow of a person's body is out of balance when there is disease. Ki flow is the life force or electromagnetic field of the body. Many things in the modern person's environment interfere with this flow of energy. The type of diet also affects Ki flow because each kind of food is a type of energy. Macrobiotic teaching defines various foods as either yin (expansive) or yang (contracting) energy. Depending on a person's health and constitution, they need to eat more yin or more yang foods or foods that are more centrally balanced between the two energies.

In addition, some types of clothing such as synthetics are said to disrupt Ki flow, whereas a natural fiber such as cotton does not. Wearing metals in the form of watches, bracelets, earrings, and necklaces also obstructs Ki flow, thereby contributing to the creation of "dis-ease" in the body. Along a similar line of consideration, canned and frozen foods lack vital Ki or life force.

When Michael and Mickey decided to adopt a macrobiotic lifestyle and approach to healing, they read and studied these principles intensely to understand them properly. Mickey said, "We went after every ounce of information we could find with a vengeance. I didn't want Michael to die. I wasn't about to let him die — I had faith that Michael was strong enough to heal himself. My faith was so strong there was no way he couldn't get better. I just wouldn't acknowledge the fact he could die."

The first couple of weeks, however, Michael said he was like a zombie. "I couldn't believe it. It makes you numb. There was blind fear. Nothing else matters. I didn't care about work or eating. I didn't care about anything. I think I lost ten pounds in a week. And I am a voracious eater. I couldn't eat. There I was fairly newly married and it was going to end like this. That's when Mickey took charge and said, 'That's not going to happen. There are ways to deal with this.' Mickey was very strong. Her attitude was, 'We are going to beat this.' She was terrific."

In spite of the fear Michael experienced at the beginning, Mickey knew he had the will and desire to survive. "We used to go for walks every night. The first two nights after learning about the melanoma, we went on our usual two-mile walk and we talked and we cried. I kept saying 'Why? It isn't fair.' I couldn't understand it; on the other hand, I was somewhat accepting that this was God's plan. I suggested we buy the book *Death and Dying*. When I said that, Michael really came back at me and asked, 'Why did you say that?' Surprised at his response, I said, 'If it's inevitable that you are going to die in six months time, I think you should read that book.' He came out of his slump and said, 'I am not doing to die.' There was something there. I just knew he was healthy and that the cancer could not consume him. He had too much willpower to buckle into it."

Mickey was encouraged by their first visit to see Lino Stanchich, a macrobiotic teacher. "The first thing he told Michael was — though Michael may have malignant melanoma — his outward appearance (based on physiognomy) was too vital to be a man who should be dead in three months. Lino confirmed my thoughts. There was no reason for him to die. I felt really positive about this. And Michael began to come around. After talking with Alan and seeing Lino, there was never a doubt in our minds that he wouldn't be well."

"We bought a gas stove immediately and had it installed in a week's time. We did a thorough housecleaning. We gave away all canned foods and threw away all the frozen food and anything that was processed or had a chemical in it. Within the first week, I cleaned out my kitchen totally. Michael removed the I.D. bracelet he had worn forever and took off his watch. His wedding ring was the only piece of metal he would wear. We threw away or gave away any item of clothing that had polyester in it, anything that was not made of natural cotton. I mean our whole world turned upside down." As Mickey characterized it, "The first couple of weeks were pretty heavy-duty."

At the same time Michael and Mickey were starting to make these changes in their lives, Michael kept getting calls from the oncologists' office. The test results were in. The oncologists wanted

Michael to go to the University of Alabama ". . . where there is a world-renowned melanoma surgeon." They told him, "We feel surgery is what you want to do. Since we can't find the primary site we will deal with the area of the original surgery, excise that to a greater degree and then probably go down into the neck . . . and maybe down into the arm and lymph nodes, depending on how advanced it might be."

"But part of the tests I had were lymph tests," Michael said. "They took samples of fluid and cells from nodes in that area and couldn't find anything. Even knowing this they still wanted to take stuff. So, I said, 'OK, I'll think about that.' I have worked with people who have gone through melanoma surgery. It's absolutely brutal. They cut everything away, huge margins and very, very deep. You lose part of your jaw. It's unbelievable. It's very mutilating. If it's going to keep you alive, wonderful. But that doesn't even work so why go through all that?

"There is a book by Jean Kohler, one of the first macrobiotic books out. Jean did not die from cancer. Doctors confirmed he died of an infection caused by prior surgery. It was a dormant infection that became active. An autopsy showed Jean Kohler did not have any cancer activity in his body . . . seven years after he was diagnosed as having pancreatic cancer. I have never been one to have surgery for the sake of having surgery.

"Finally, I got a registered, return-receipt letter from the West Palm Beach oncologist dated April 4, 1985, telling me that if I didn't have the operation, I would die. He wrote: 'Dear Mr. Shanik: As you are aware, the melanoma of the right scalp, from which you presently suffer has been in my opinion as well as that of other physicians inadequately treated to date. Further conventional therapy, including evaluation for extent of lymphatic drainage and metastasis as well as an excision of this region is recommended. If you refuse to follow through with these recommendations, it is most likely that the disease will reoccur locally, in other words, in the right scalp and/or metastasize (spread) to other parts of the body and would result in your death from what may well be a curable situation. It is important that you understand the seriousness of this situation. I'm sure you understand the options as we discussed them in the past.

Many times people accept unconventional therapy because they just can't quite accept the fact that they really have such a threatening form of cancer. If there is anything I can do to help direct you in a way that can salvage this situation, I'll be happy to meet with you at anytime or speak to you on the phone, but I need for you to be aware of the high risk you're taking by choosing your present course of action, which appears limited to using a macrobiotic diet. I trust that I have made myself clear.'"

"That letter was quite a test for me. It was like receiving a death notice. That's exactly what it felt like. In the meantime, we had met other macrobiotic people at the Foundation who had been dealing with melanoma. I called them to find out what to do. Of course, nobody can make those kinds of decisions for you, and they didn't attempt to make them either. They said, "You just have to weigh what you believe in." I had read so much about surgery being so invasive. I finally decided against it and that was that. I believed macrobiotics was going to work. From an energy aspect, I started feeling better. The philosophy of macrobiotics and the case after case that I read of people who made themselves well just made sense to me. The current statistics of 10 to 20 percent survival rate are very, very dismal. If the statistics had been different, probably it would have been a different story. The only time the statistics are fairly favorable with melanoma is if they find the primary site fairly early and it hasn't moved. Say it's a mole or something on your body and you are suspicious of it. They test it for melanoma, it's positive and the mole is removed rather deeply. People who have that kind of surgery fair quite well."

March 22, 1985, two weeks before he received the letter from the doctor, Michael and Mickey went to Boston where they attended a Way of Life Seminar for beginners in macrobiotics on how to apply macrobiotic principles to their diet and daily life. They attended this seminar before meeting with Michio Kushi. "I think the orientation was two or three days," said Michael. "There were probably forty of fifty people in the class. They had cooking classes and lectures on the philosophy. All the foods were there on the table, the different kinds of beans and grains, vegetables and seaweeds. Michio, Edward Esko and Marc Van Cauwenberghe lectured. Evelyne

Harboun, a Moroccan woman, demonstrated how to prepare ginger compresses and other home care. It was very thorough. The program was from morning until evening for three solid days. The orientation was extremely important to us."

"We had a month's time from when we saw Lino in Miami," Mickey recalls, "until we went to Boston. In that one month we learned an awful lot about macrobiotics. By the time we got back from Boston we were very knowledgeable as to what macrobiotics was and what to do. We followed this diet religiously." As a consequence, both Michael and Mickey were well informed about macrobiotics and practicing it diligently when the doctor's letter arrrived.

In June, 1985, Michael went for a second interview with Mr. Kushi. "Mickey was with me and we brought Christopher with us to meet Michael. Meeting with Michio is always wonderful. We chatted with Michio at the beginning. After observing my condition, Michio said, 'It seems you have turned the corner with your illness. You are well on the way to recovery.'

"Mickey and I just looked at each other and almost burst into tears. We couldn't believe it was that fast. It was only four months. It was really an emotional experience. We went out and had a beer to celebrate. There was a lot of joy. I knew something was happening. I was feeling great by June. It was incredible. I just kept feeling better and better." Michael's visit to a holistic, medical doctor in September 1985 confirmed what Michio told Michael. Michael's next visit to one of his original oncologists, however, was not until February 1986, the anniversary of the original diagnosis. This doctor, practicing in Ft. Lauderdale, wrote a follow-up letter at Michael's request and attached a copy of the lab results of blood tests conducted on blood taken during the exam. This letter reads, "To Whom It May Concern: Mr. Michael Shanik was seen yesterday in this office. It has been about a year since he had resection of a metastatic node from the malignant melanoma, primary site unknown. No further local, regional or adjuvant systemic therapy was done at that time.

"He is doing very well. He appears healthy, mentally and physically. He has lost about thirty pounds with a macrobiotic diet. It seems that this approach has helped him cope very well with his physical and mental status.

"No further treatment is advised at this point, but he is urged to have medical check-ups no longer than six months apart. A complete profile, CBC and CEA were obtained. The results are not available as yet." When the results did come in, they showed the CBC and CEA were all in a normal range.

Especially significant was the examination Michael had six months later on August 29, 1986, with the oncologist in West Palm Beach who sent Michael the registered letter, the one telling Michael he would die if he did not have the recommended surgery. At Michael's request, the doctors wrote a letter dated October 7, 1986, and reporting the results of that examination, written in strictly clinical terms, its contents were as follows:

RE: Michael Shanik
Office Visit of 8-29-86

S. No pain. Appetite is good. Diet is 100 percent macrobiotic.

Fully active. Has changed his whole life to decrease stress.

Feels well.

O. Vital signs are stable. Weight 171. WBC 7.4, Hct. 43.6, Hgb. 15.6, platelets 180,000. Fundi benign. Right scalp without nodules. Chest wall is clear. Heart and lungs are normal. No abdominal masses or hepatosplenomegaly. Skin is without lesions. No lymphadenopathy. No lower extremity edema. Neurologically intact. SMA-25 was normal.

A. No evidence of palpable disease.

P. Return in six months. Call if any nodules develop.

Describing the doctors reaction on the occasion of that appointment, Michael said, "He was totally flabbergasted. He couldn't believe how I had changed and how well I was."

Prior to meeting Michael and learning about macrobiotics, Mickey was a long time frequenter of health food stores because of her interest in nutrition and natural approaches to maintaining health. In addition, she said, "I always wanted to be vegetarian because of my distaste for animals being slaughtered." Her first impressions of the primarily vegetarian macrobiotic basic diet were favorable because of this interest. Cooking macrobiotically was really attractive to her "probably because I was my closest to becoming vegetarian when I met Michael. Michael, however, introduced me to sipping a glass of sherry after dinner and having an excellent cut of meat from time to time because he felt I needed it for the blood quality. When we met, I fell away from vegetarianism. Then I gradually started climbing back again and bringing him with me. This meant eating less meat and fat plus getting him to exercise more." Michael agreed, "Mickey got me to eating a whole lot healthier than I was before, but I was by no stretch a vegetarian."

When Mickey's friend first told her about macrobiotics, he gave her some printed material about it from the Macrobiotic Foundation in Garden Grove. He also suggested she and Michael come to one of the Thursday night dinners. "I looked at the papers. It discussed the lifestyle . . . going to bed at sundown, getting up at sun up, no dairy, no meat, no alcohol, no tobacco, no this, no that." I thought, "It's much too strict. I could probably adhere to most of it, but Michael, on the other hand, would not do it at all."

When Michael and Mickey learned he had cancer, however, Mickey said, "I knew modern medicine couldn't do anything for him. They had no answers, so why not look elsewhere? The thing I had to draw upon was macrobiotics." Looking at the evidence in all the books they studied, Michael also realized this was his only real chance for survival. "The thing that impressed me the most was how scientific the writings were. Everything was discussed in chemical terms as far as how the mechanics of the food works. Somebody had done their homework and thought out how segments of food effect the body and why you get well when you eat this way. It was clear to me why it was going to work. This wasn't just some kind of voodoo with sharks' teeth. This was real."

Contrary to Mickey's impression about how Michael would react to macrobiotics, he said, "I looked at it as something that could help me. I was not suspect of it or counter to it in anyway. I can't explain why. It was as if something inside of me knew this was going to work."

Regarding his first impressions of the Miami Macrobiotic Foundation, Michael commented, "From day one it had a very nice feel about it. The building is nice and the people have a nice way about them Basically, it's one large room separated into a dining room, small office, reception area, and counselor's office . . . very plain, austere . . . like the dining hall at a summer camp with exposed beams, white wall, wooden floors, nothing fancy. There's so much going on there it's terribly crowded. It's not uncommon for them to get eighty people for a dinner: the center is growing like crazy. But it's a good facility and good people." Michael especially enjoyed the diverse interests of the people who came to the center.

Most important of all, however, was his response to macrobiotic food. "I love all of it." And whereas Mickey admits, "Seaweed took some getting used to. It was just too fishy and strong for me," she adds, "Michael liked it immediately . . . but then Michael likes everything. That's why it was so easy. Michael likes to eat and I like to cook. Everything I made, he thought was truly wonderful. And that was always ten points for my ego. The more he jumped up and down and loved the food, and the better he looked, the more I cooked." Consequently, both say the transition to eating macrobiotically was not difficult for them. Mickey says it was easy for her because "I was basically always wanting to cook more naturally anyway." Michael attributes the ease of his transition to Mickey. "Since I'm married to such a phenomenal cook the food is so interesting. She's very innovative. It's never the same. And if it is the same dish, it tastes different than the prior time." The toughest thing for Michael to master was learning how to chew. You're supposed to chew each mouthful fifty to one hundred times. It took constant reminding and a lot of indigestion before I disciplined myself to do this. Lino was very persistent, very much like a Prussian general. It finally dawned on me that chewing has an integral part in the benefit one receives from the food. According to macrobiotics, a good portion of digestion occurs in the mouth."

Regarding the Japanese terms and names of some of the foods, Michael recalled having difficulty with these at the beginning. "But you get used to it. Our kitchen set up is so different. Once you get oriented, those are the ingredients you use. Also, you have all these whole foods and are a lot more involved with it. These are dried foods in jars that you have to make sure don't get bugs. You refrigerate so much here in Florida because it's so buggy, and bugs that come in foods germinate. Refrigeration is critical to fresh produce. You don't have cans you place on the shelves or frozen foods to fill the freezer. The refrigerator in the kitchen has no freezer. The freezer is out in the garage and it's very small. Whereas before I might go to the store once a week, maybe twice, now I'm there four and five times for fresh produce. That's half the diet and it has to be fresh. But again, you get used to it." In fact, Michael admits he likes this involvement. Having to buy and eat foods only when they are fresh and in season puts him in touch with nature in a very direct way that he didn't experience before. "This may sound poetic and mushy, but it creates a sense of oneness with the universe," an awareness that he said enriches his life daily.

Though the transition went relatively smoothly for them both, Mickey said, "I was real nervous in the beginning. I burned the first pot of brown rice the night we got home from the health food store. I thought, "Oh, my god! His life really depends on my ability to cook right for him! I knew it wasn't a forever thing, but it was critical at that point in time. I knew his problems were being taken care of by macrobiotics and by God, but I had a part to play and that was being the cook. As I got used to it, everything got easier. Also, my kids were great and very supportive of macrobiotics. We used to eat at health food stores when we were in Michigan and there were just the three of us. When they were six and seven, I used to make 'Tofu Surprise' dinners for them and they would go 'Oh, no, what has she done this time?' They always figured I was a little crazy." When she started macrobiotic cooking, Mickey said, "I was nervous with them because they didn't like everything. Their tastes were so jaded from eating junk at school and with their friends. If you eat a frozen, sugary slurpy, it's very difficult to find flavor in a simple bowl of brown rice. For that reason, not too many things were very tasty for them. I was cooking almost a separate meal for Christopher. Andrea would eat with Michael and me. That got old after about four or five months. I was finding it pretty difficult and I started having Christopher eat with us. If he didn't like what we were eating, he was more than able to go into the kitchen and make a peanut butter and jelly sandwich if that's what he wanted."

"From the beginning, though, my kids really showed they cared a great deal for Michael and were concerned with his welfare; they wanted him to be well. Michael has no children of his own. He really appreciated the thought that he had a family at the time. His own family is gone so my family is his family. They are part of a good reason to continue being here. There were people who needed him." About her mother and other relatives, she said, "None of my family is macrobiotic. Some don't even understand it, but they have been very supportive. No one has ever put us down. These are all people in Wisconsin dairyland. Even strangers thought it was commendable."

Generally, Michael has had a similar experience. Always pretty much of a loner, he never conducted much business over lunch or maintained an extensive social life so there has not been much conflict resulting in his change from eating a mainstream American diet to macrobiotics.

"When I was working for this design firm," Michael recalls, "there was one instance, however, where I brought my lunch. Everybody went out to lunch and I had my little tin of food and I ate from that. The feedback I got was that my boss was very uncomfortable with that. I didn't say anything but I avoided going out to lunch anymore. Nowadays, we will take a customer to a health food restaurant and since I am eating wider, I know what to order in a restaurant. I can have pasta or salad or something like that. But we don't entertain people a lot. Neither of us do.

"Eating white flour pasta one time won't hurt me. It's like eating white rice. When we go to a Japanese restaurant, very few of them have brown rice. We have Kappa-Sushi. I won't eat sushi rice because it usually has sugar in it. I request plain white rice. It doesn't have a lot of food value, but it isn't harmful. It's the same with white flour pasta. Usually, better Italian restaurants will use natural flour pasta like semolina or durum wheat anyway. I have a little olive oil and garlic on it. Then, every year when we go to Chicago, we have to eat at a fancy restaurant called Chez Joseph with a group of people who represent this one company.

"The first year, Mickey and I were the only ones who were vegetarian. Usually better restaurants will make a plate for you . . . steamed vegetables and rice or whatever. This year there were five of us at the table eating the same thing. So it's changed. It was a surprise to the restaurant. It was not a problem for them at all. If we are worried about it, we call ahead so the restaurant can get vegetables in, but they always have broccoli, cauliflower, beans or something like that . . . enough to survive on and go through the ceremony."

Since the time Michael was diagnosed as having cancer and throughout the initial recovery period, he continued to work. "I didn't feel bad or have symptoms like some people do when they have cancer. Since I had no medical treatment other than minor surgery, I didn't have devastating symptoms from that.

"I didn't travel much, I can tell you that. At the time I was diagnosed, I was doing marketing for a design firm in Fort Lauderdale. I was selling their service. They were interior designers for developers and people like that who need a design firm. So I traveled the local area. I didn't have long distance trips Then we started our own business Mickey started it and then I joined her a year later. Our business now requires that we travel, but in the two years I was on the healing diet, I traveled very little. I was advised by the (macrobiotic) counselors not to. They tell you to stay close to home. 'Be more in control of what you eat; you can't afford to eat that widely when you are on a healing diet.'

"Now we are traveling more. We have a Minneapolis trip coming up then on to New Mexico, Arizona and Toronto. But, we have already made our arrangements. We call ahead for food and lodging. I know where all the health food stores and restaurants are and where there are people who serve macrobiotic food in their home. We will have trouble finding appropriate food in the Grand Canyon area. There I will buy a gas camping stove and a little pot. We will take dried ingredients with us in our suitcases. I will buy fresh produce and cook in our room." With a touch of irony in his voice, Michael added, "One of my greatest fantasies is that all the restaurants in the country are macrobiotic and the odd restaurants are the ones that serve standard Western food . . . beef, etc. And, you have to seek those out or call ahead so they can slaughter a cow for you and things like that. All the other restaurants would be like Five Seasons or Open Sesame (popular macrobiotic restaurants in the Boston area near the Kushi Institute). He added somewhat wistfully, "It would be nice to go up to the Grand Canyon to a little stand and be served tofu and things like that." Nevertheless, in spite of the obstacles, Michael and Mickey take this all in their stride and manage the situation in the elegant style typical of them.

Michael took time and reflected on the dietary causes of his cancer. "I would say my downfall was dairy. I loved cheese." He also thinks he was bottle fed as an infant. As a child he said, "I liked everything. Foodwise, I was easy to satisfy. We were a typical middle class family in the forties and fifties. That meant pot roast, chicken and usually meat at every evening meal . . . also fish. There was lots of dairy food because of the family history. They were dairy farmers. And I always ate to excess, always. I was never obese. I was big, but I lost a lot of weight in the military. I was in very good shape, but I was a glutton. Anything I ate, I ate too much of. No discipline at all. Then I would go on diets. If a diet was faddish — such as the Atkins Diet — I would do it. Then I would gain it all back. It was tough to keep the weight off. I resigned myself to it. I figured at my age you just accumulate weight and it was going to stay on period." Though salads were always a favorite food, he said, "I usually covered it with blue cheese dressing or something like that." In addition to cheese and salads Michael said, "I loved breads and pasta. Fortunately, I can have pasta and a little bit of bread. But it hasn't been hard to be macrobiotic because the foods are so wonderful."

When Michael started macrobiotics he weighed 200 lbs. In four months time he weighed 155. I'm 5'11". I was bigger than I should be, big enough to where bending over to tie my shoes made me breathe hard. But I was also very physically active. We rode bikes and everything. I just ate the wrong things and too much." With the weight loss during the initial healing stage when he began macrobiotics, he observed other changes. "I would say within two weeks I felt completely different. In reading, I found your blood quality changes very quickly and that makes a profound difference.

There was one moment when I was on a call at a college. It was a large meeting and I remember I could not recall ever thinking so clearly. That was early in mid-March. Usually at things like that I tend to drift away into my own thoughts. I don't pay a lot of attention because it's kind of boring. It was a very dull group and a dull subject. Nevertheless, there were some decisions that had to be made. My pitch was an important part for insuring our firm's participation and I was very sharp at that. Generally, I have noticed I am much sharper in my thinking. Before then, I felt at forty-four you are getting older and your thoughts get a little dimmer. Your body is a lot more sluggish. That is not the way it has to be at all though. I have a lot more energy, too."

Whereas Michael experienced having more energy, after several months of eating macrobiotically, Mickey felt she didn't have enough. "I was feeling a little bit heavy. More than likely we were eating too much grain. We were not eating for the climate here. We were following more of a Boston diet and not one for Florida. About this same time, she and Michael considered other approaches besides macrobiotics. One program that appealed to both Michael and Mickey was one advocated by Bernard Jensen, a Naturopathic doctor, chiropractor and leading proponent of iridology. The raw foods component of Jensen's holistic healing approach was especially attractive to Michael and Mickey. Alan Jacobs, who originally inspired Michael to give macrobiotics a try, was going to an iridologist versed in the Jensen program. "We wanted to lighten up," Michael recalled, "so we started going to the same guy as Alan. The raw foods were wonderful. In macrobiotics nearly everything is cooked. With the raw foods, there wasn't much food preparation or cooking involved. They were cooler, but also harder to digest. But we weren't on the track very long. Also involved were colonics and I had two that I thought were going to kill me. I wound up with a killer case of hemorrhoids so bad I was in terrible pain for about two or three months. The pain was unbelievable. I wouldn't take any drugs either. We used all kinds of poultices, packs and suppositories and finally just time to make it better. Mickey took the colonics fine. She was okay, but I am just not built to handle it. That was part of the regimen for internal cleansing. This makes some sense, but it's also not real natural to be hosing out your behind all the time. Macrobiotics cleanses the system too, but it's not extreme in anyway. It is easy on the body, so it works."

Besides the discomfort Michael experienced with the raw foods and colonics program, he and Mickey were alarmed by the effects it had upon their friend, Alan. Mickey explained, "When we looked at this colonic thing, cleaning out the intestines made sense to me, too. If we eat wrong for so many years, I am sure we get very clogged up. If you think about it, when you clean that stuff out of there you have better absorption of nutrients and minerals you are taking in. I thought if Alan is doing it and he's feeling better, which he was, that might be good for us since we were feeling sluggish. Well, Michael had such a rough time with it that he couldn't do it, and we watched our friend start to deteriorate. Alan peaked in a couple of weeks after starting the raw foods and citrus. Then he started going down hill." During this period Michael and Mickey didn't go off their macrobiotic diet entirely, however. Said Mickey, "We were only dabbling with it a little bit. We were still eating our miso soup and seaweeds, but for breakfast I maybe just had citrus instead of sitting down to grains and miso soup. I was half macrobiotic and half doing fruits, taking herbs and having colonics. Once we saw Alan deteriorate, he just went so fast. I got scared. I thought, "Oh no. If it happened this fast with him, what in the world is going on inside Michael right now." So I called Lino. I was very afraid for Michael. I told Lino the whole story."

Michael remembered Lino's response. "He said, 'I will tell you why. It didn't have to happen. He ate much too widely and threw his body out of balance.'" Mickey commented on the healing approach the iridologist was using. "It wasn't a macrobiotic thought process, (i.e. based on yin and yang energy concept). I look at macrobiotics as being the basics. Once you are macrobiotic any length of time, it starts becoming natural to think in those terms. After talking to Lino I went back to a macrobiotic breakfast, lunch and dinner, no deviating, no nothing. I felt like I came back to where I belonged."

Since that time they have not tried any other natural healing programs. "The only thing I have done," said Mickey, "is align our diet and cooking with Florida weather and seasons. Mickey has also adjusted the diet to meet her own particular needs. "When we started macrobiotics, I ate the same diet as Michael, and I ended up very, very yang or tight. I did not have periods. I was tense and kind of snappy if I was tired. So I went to Lino and he suggested a few things for me that Michael couldn't go near."

The foods suggested by Lino are considered more yin or expansive in energy. Melanoma, however, is a condition requiring the individual who has it to eat foods that are neither extremely yin or extremely yang in energy, but are a natural balance of the two. Though not precisely corresponding with yin and yang, the Western concept of pH balance is similar when considering the biochemistry of the human body and other organic systems such as plants, for instance. It's important for the human body to maintain a slightly alkaline condition to be able to efficiently metabolize food and "burn" it cleanly. If the body takes in foods that are too acidic, a condition called acidosis occurs. The opposite occurs when we take in foods that are primarily alkaline. When this happens we are prone to "disease." Certain plants, for example, require an acid soil to grow and develop properly whereas others require an alkaline or neutral soil. If conditions of the soil are other than that required, full growth and health potential is impaired. This same principle applies to the human body. The concept of yin and yang operates similarly, only here the emphasis is based on the type of energy rather than chemical balance. Given the difference in condition and makeup of Mickey's body as contrasted with Michael's, she required more "yin" energy foods. Weather also affects what types of food energy the body requires. Hot weather increases the need for more yin type foods. Cold weather, on the other hand, sees an increased need for more yang.

"We see Lino formally every seasonal change, four times a year and he advises us how to readjust the diet," said Michael. Also, as his health has improved, Michael pointed out that Michio and macrobiotic counselors never put themselves up as any cure-all. "They weren't going to make me well. Mickey and I were going to make me well. Everything points back to you. You are going to do this. The litany throughout macrobiotic philosophy is that you are responsible. You are responsible for (creating) disease and you are responsible for (creating) wellness. You are in charge. That appeals to me."

Concerning the economics of macrobiotics, Michael observed, "Whole food costs less than processed foods. We are eating grains, beans, and vegetables as opposed to meats which are expensive. Also, we hardly eat out anymore. So that cost dropped dramatically. I think the initial set up was $1,000, with the gas stove, all the equipment we needed and the initial food. But when it comes to your life, so what? The cost factor never entered into our decision. Compared to any medical therapy, even with what you pay out of your pocket, including the initial educational programs, it's far less money. At the time, I never thought about that, but this is what we are going to do, whatever it costs."

Mickey agrees that initially their food costs dropped by a third. Since she tends to cook a gourmet style, however, there are many non-essential, but acceptable ingredients that are more expensive. In that case, "It's about the same cost if you were eating a usual modern diet. Japanese specialty food items such as chestnut paste, umeboshi plums, etc. cost more than if one sticks to macrobiotic basics." However, she added, "You can put together some absolutely incredible dinners using these wonderful ingredients. To be creative with food — this is the fun of it."

Eating out at a macrobiotic restaurant is another matter altogether. "Michael and I used to spend $250 a month eating out and those were just quicky dinners at the deli. If we ate an expensive dinner it would end up being $150, $175, which is totally absurd. Now we have wonderful gourmet dinners in a New York macrobiotic restaurant and walk out of there having spent $25 or $30. It's great. Your values change." Mickey will confess, however, to missing an occasional dinner in the ambiance of "little, sexy French cafes" or "having a piece of cheesecake." "Nevertheless, she also says, "I miss that but not to the point where I would eat it. I cheated a little bit by eating a piece of chocolate cake and I had a peach melba sundae once, but I didn't feel well afterwards." She recognizes the low quality of these foods and that they do not contribute "to my health and well being. You just have to change your headset. It's a different lifestyle."

Speaking of these changes in lifestyle, Michael said about macrobiotics, "I think for anybody who has gone through a life-threatening illness, the discipline is much greater. I didn't have any choice. But it has opened up so many things in my life. The food is really a minor, though very important, part. I am a totally different person than I used to be. I was much more hyper . . . very much a Type A person. I have calmed down a lot. People who knew me before can't believe the difference. Not that I don't have my moments. Everyone does." Michael elaborated, "I was much more driven. I had to work. I had to push. Now I don't feel I have to push so much. And, now that I don't have to, I'm doing better with the business." Regarding Type A, he said, "I don't think I have that mentality anymore. I would make more money, but I don't need any more money. For what? I never had the killer instinct about money. I worked hard. We had what we wanted, but how much can you want?" Michael also described himself as being more job-oriented before his cancer diagnosis. "My job was fun and we had a good time with it, but it's not everything. I would rather ride my bike and do other things." How he reacts to pressure has changed as well. "Knowing what I know now, life's little problems are even smaller. I used to get whacked out about very minor things, trivial things and I don't anymore. In business, it's one thing after another . . . something breaking or getting screwed up. Clients get upset because you aren't upset enough about these things. But it's not important enough to upset your own harmony. A little stress is good for you. It's a kind of prod that keeps you going. But I think a harmonious family and work situation is very important to your health. Too much anxiety is detrimental. It absolutely erodes your health."

Michael and Mickey now live on the west coast of Florida where they moved about a year after learning he had cancer. In addition to the pond and wildlife in the back of their house, to the side and front is a pool and well maintained lawn screened by a thick wall of native bushes, trees and plants. A private beach shared by other residents of Sandy Hook Road is a five-minute walk from Michael and Mickey's house and offers a sweeping panorama of the Gulf of Mexico. "My appreciation for things around me has increased. I think that is part of the reason we are living over here. It has more natural surroundings than the other side of the state. I always did have a love of and an interest in nature, but it's more keen now."

"I also think our business has improved in that our attitude is much calmer. Our business doubled last year and will probably double again this year. Good things just tend to happen to us. They really do. Whatever waves you send out, you get back. I really believe that. We are in more control. Number one, we have our own business, so we call the shots as opposed to working for somebody else. We come and go when we want, but we have a sense of responsibility toward our business. There are a lot of things that are going on which I like. I like variety. I could never sit idle."

"There's more than one way to deal with disease, but with macrobiotics, it's not just a fix. It becomes more of a way of life. There are so many other things so totally enchancing to your life that comes with macrobiotics. The people it has brought us in touch with are tremendous; for example, the people we met through the (macrobiotic) Foundations in Boston and Miami. Also, there are the people I met and have tried to help or read stories about and called."

An important aspect of a person's healing is regaining balance of Ki within oneself and with the universe around and beyond oneself. Consequently, individuals studying macrobiotic principles are encouraged to delve into and become actively involved in spiritual practices of their ancestors or a tradition that feels right to them.

Previously unconcerned about this aspect of life, Michael's close encounter with death definitely has affected his outlook on spiritual matters. Raised Jewish, Michael said he was Bar Mizvahed at thirteen and attended Hebrew school for five or six years. "And that was the end of it. I was forced to go to Hebrew School. It was what one did. I didn't look at that training as having any relationship to anything." Recently, however, he met some Orthodox Jews, has become interested in the Talmud and would like to join a study group, but does not want to get involved in a synagogue. In addition, he has expressed an interest in learning more about Buddhism and exploring Native American spirituality. In general, he says he attributes more importance to spiritual growth than before and looks forward to attending Michio Kushi's seminar on spirituality when he and Mickey are able to. On the other hand, Mickey said about spiritual growth, "I have always been looking and seeking, especially since I was twenty-seven or twenty-eight . . . one group after another. Nothing has been right for me. The most right thing has been sitting in a tree or sitting outside on the ground. If anything I am looking into my own thoughts on religion which are earth-centered. If I looked into our native American customs and ways of belief, I am sure that is where I would end up."

Nurturing a grateful heart and attitude is also an important part of obtaining and maintaining balance and right relationship with Ki or life force. Said Mickey of hers and Michael's own spiritual quest, "We both are so very grateful for all our blessings; we would like to make sure we are thanking someone properly."

Among the many other changes Michael has experienced he says, "Family is much more important to me now. Needless to say, that's Mickey's because mine is all gone. They are all pretty good folks and we spend a lot of time with them. Before, we might have chosen to do something else in lieu of doing that. I encourage Mickey to visit them. She's very close with her grandfather who's ninety-eight or ninety-nine and lives in Wisconsin. She's lucky to have him. I think you have more of an appreciation for those ties. You realize how grateful you are for being alive. All aspects of your life are more highly tuned so you nurture them, whereas before you might have been more cavalier and that's wrong." Michael's own mother died of cancer at age fifty-seven. His sister was age forty-six when she, too, died of cancer. Michael was there with them both throughout their illnesses.

Today, a primary concern of Michael's is to share with others what he has learned about the benefits of macrobiotics. Speaking of the registered letter he received from his doctor, he said, "I don't need someone else to tell me I feel good. I know my blood is normal. If it wasn't, I'd feel it. I go to the doctors for the letters. I want a high stack, and ten years from now I still hope to be talking to people. I was at one seminar and there were a couple of people in the audience who wanted to see these letters and the blood workups attached to them. Seeing that absolutely turned them around. Rather than just a testimonial, here was evidence. That means an awful lot to people."

Michael plans to continue practicing macrobiotics "pretty strictly" from the food aspect, and as far as doing for others, he helps people wherever he can, on the phone or speaking, whatever he can do to assist them in getting acclimated to it. Mickey and he also have started Gray Dove Inn, a macrobiotic bed and breakfast in their guest house. The guest house is an offshoot of part of what we wanted to give back to macrobiotics," he explained, "thereby providing a place for macrobiotic people (primarily) to come, vacation and enjoy themselves." About what his future plans are involving macrobiotics, Michael added, "I am exploring a possible opportunity in the health food field. Whether it comes to pass or not I don't know. That would be a complete career change. "In addition, he and Mickey are taking a nine-month long, intensive macrobiotic study program one weekend a month in Miami. "We need to know a lot more than we do about food and philosophy for self-improvement and self-knowledge.

"Macrobiotics is attracting more mainstream people. There are a lot of professional people in it. A number of lawyers, accountants, and consultants are involved in the Foundation in Miami. It's good to see that happening. Mainstream people will influence other mainstream people in the mass of society. The way we change things is by example, by the people we associate with, people, for instance, who come into this house.

"I was very much a crusader. I was going to change everybody. I was hard selling. But that stopped. I still take the initiative to call somebody and see if I can help them, but once I get resistance, I stop. That's it. I mention it to them. I don't paint an unrealistic picture. If people see you are healthy, that you are walking around and know what you had, they have to add two and two together.

"Mickey is starting a cooking class for a lady we have met here on the island. There are friends who are going to become involved. We will probably have six or eight people at that cooking class who won't even know how to spell macrobiotics. If anything will happen, at least they will be conscious of better eating and how important that is to their general health."

Mickey looked back over all the changes they both have undergone since the cancer diagnosis. Considering her longstanding interest in health, natural foods and vegetarianism, she concluded, "It's almost like it was time for Michael to get sick so I could make my transition. We came together for a particular reason. I wasn't ready to let go of him then. I feel there is more for us to do together. Now he has a real cause and that's to be an example to people."

As for how she is different, Mickey said, "Before, I would go to someone and say, 'You should do this,' whereas now, I am much more gentle. If I have an approach on something, I don't push it on people. I'm not as pushy . . . I am a much nicer person. And I have learned so many things."

About Michael she said, "He is a different person. It's almost as if he died and started all over. He had a wonderful opportunity. After our first trips to Boston, we were saying it was a blessing. Michael said cancer was the best thing that happened to him."

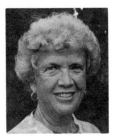

3

Phyllis Crabtree
Uterine and Breast Cancer

The startling news that she had uterine cancer caught Phyllis Crabtree mid-stride a full and active life. It was October 1972. Phyllis was director of day nursery for low-income, disadvantaged children and also just beginning to teach a college level course in special education at Pennsylvania State University. At age fifty, she was mother of two adult children in their twenties and wife to Allen Crabtree, a prominent local businessman in State College, Pennsylvania. In addition to civic and church involvements, when needed, Phyllis sometimes also helped out in her husband's jewelry store, a store started by Allen Crabtree's father.

Within two-and-a-half months after learning of the uterine cancer, Phyllis underwent two operations. During the first one in October, 1972, Phyllis' uterus, ovaries and fallopian tubes were removed. As a result of subsequent tests on December 31, 1972, the doctor informed her she had breast cancer as well. The very next day, New Year's Day, 1973, Phyllis' right breast was surgically removed during a radical mastectomy. Statistics available to her at the time indicated only fifteen out of a hundred women who had these two cancer operations in sequence would be alive five years later.

Faced with the reality of these hard statistics, Phyllis was thrust into a great fear for her life. To improve her chances for survival and at the insistence of her son, Phil, Phyllis began to carefully choose, eat and prepare her food according to macrobiotic dietary principles. To avoid the debilitating side effects of radiation and chemotherapy, she also refused further standard medical treatment recommended to her. In these decisions she had the wholehearted and loving support of her husband, Allen.

Today, nineteen years later, Phyllis is a cheerful, active, outgoing woman in her sixties. An avid grandmother and traveler, she is grateful for restored health and the security she gains from continuing to eat macrobiotically. Both Phyllis and her husband are retired now and enjoy taking trips in their camper, hiking in the mountains and waterskiing.

Prior to the cancer diagnosis and before starting to eat macrobiotically, she was plagued with chronic bladder infections, hemorrhoids, migraine headaches, and osteoporosis. Phyllis' daughter, Kathy, who lives in Ontario, Canada, recalls a childhood during which her mother was "always sick with something." Kathy is pleased to report her mother is "never sick now." Phyllis' son, Phil, also proudly tells how, on a visit to see him in Washington State, his mother climbed to the snow line of Mt. Rainier.

Born, raised and educated in State College, Pennsylvania, hometown of Pennsylvania State University, Phyllis married Allen Crabtree, her high school sweetheart, in 1943. The marriage took place shortly after Phyllis graduated from Penn State and just before Allen, then a young Army officer, was sent off to Europe during World War II. Graduating with highest marks in her department, Phyllis' course of study was pre-med. Her career goal was to be a medical doctor. Before Allen left for overseas, however, Phyllis found she was pregnant. Consequently, her plans took a new direction. A couple of years after daughter Kathy was born, Phyllis gave birth to her son, Phil. Phyllis was homemaker and mother during the growing up years of her daughter and son. Twenty-five years after receiving her bachelor's degree, Phyllis earned a Master's of Education degree in Child Development and Family Relationships. She spent twenty years as director of the day nursery before retiring in

1981.

Though independent and forthright in manner and sometimes considered a maverick in thought and action (by her own admission), Phyllis Crabtree describes her lifestyle as socially conservative and conventional. Family, church and community are central to her life and who she is as a person as well as a Christian. Representing only a quick cross-section of her many endeavors, Phyllis is a member of long standing in a Presbyterian church, has taught Sunday school since her youth, holds a twenty-five year badge from the Brownies and currently is a member of the Women's League of Voters. She lives today in the same handsome but modest home she and Allen built shortly after his return from the war. A modern house in design, it is heated primarily with wood that Allen cuts himself and brings down from nearby mountains.

It was January 1987 when Phyllis was interviewed for this story. Wide glass picture windows of the Crabtree's living room and dining area framed a snow-covered backyard bordered by dark green hemlock fir and leaf-bare hardwood trees. The strong presence of outdoors and nature flowed into Phyllis' comfortable living room. On pine-panelled walls, over the fire place and nearby pinewood book shelves were photographic portraits of early nineteenth century and Civil War era ancestors. The room held a timeless sense of connection with nature and many preceding generations. In this pleasant atmosphere and surrounded by more recent family momentos, Phyllis spoke with candor and openness about her encounter with cancer and involvement with macrobiotics. Her story, to be told in proper context, is the continuing story of an American family also touched by the turmoil and controversy of the Vietnam era. Torn by the complex issues of that time, hers is the story of how the Crabtree family came together again in spite of differences with bonds rebuilt and strengthened in the face of enormous personal adversity.

"At the time, for me, cancer was just about synonymous with death. It was like someone saying, 'You have cancer. We will operate, but you will probably die very soon.' I thought, 'Not me. No, I don't have cancer. I'm too young to die. I'm not through living yet.'" Phyllis originally went to the doctor thinking she was having problems usually associated with her age — irregular period, etc. However, "a D&C [dilatation and curettage] and biopsy on October 11 revealed there were tissues present which were termed 'precancerous.'" Phyllis and her husband were assured by the doctor that a hysterectomy was relatively routine. Because the operation presumed to be "getting it out early" Allen said, "I felt reasonably sure it was going to work out all right." Phyllis, on the other hand, was not so sure. Receiving little information from the doctor, she researched the subject herself. After reading as many articles as she could find on women and hysterectomies, she concluded this operation was "the most unnecessary operation in surgery. . . ." Before receiving the results of the doctor's tests, she wrote him and said she did not want a hysterectomy unless she had a second and third opinion. All three opinions had to be in agreement as to the need for it. In response the doctor sent her a letter. Phyllis said, "He requested I go elsewhere for future gynecological care." She was relieved to learn the frozen tissue section taken in the biopsy produced negative results and was not concerned about the doctor's reaction. Several days later, however (after results from more thorough tests were in) her doctor called to tell her she had "atypical endometrial hyperplasia." He told her this was a form of cancer and urged immediate surgery. Confronted with this frightening reality and the very real potential of her own death, she was forced to make a hard decision. The decision was made all the more difficult considering the disagreement between her and the doctor over the need for a second and third opinion. "I live in a small town. The only other gynecological service was a team, one of whom I did not care for. As I saw it I had three choices. I could go to the local hospital, swallow my pride and ask my gynecologist to do the surgery. Or I could go to one of two other hospitals outside of town. I chose the first option. Phil was around then saying there were other options, but at that time I did not believe a diet could help my condition. My reaction was, 'You do what your doctor says.' She tried to postpone the operation so it would not interupt the course she was teaching, but she finally agreed with the doctor to go into the hospital as soon as a bed was available.

The preceding year, 1972, was stressful for Phyllis. During the weeks of tests that culminated in the hysterectomy, her father suffered several strokes. These affected the use of his muscles and power of reasoning. Earlier in the year there was a fire in her kitchen, and in the summer, hurricane Agnes left sixteen inches of water in her family room. To top all this, the toughest thing she says she had to do was to tell her mother she had cancer. To explain her feelings about this experience she shared the following. "The Japanese definition of happiness is, 'Grandparents die, parents die, children die' — the idea being it's horrible to see one's own children or grandchildren die." She did not want to bring this sorrow to her mother.

There was a positive side to the picture, however. Several years of discord for Phyllis and Allen between them and their own children had begun to dissolve. Both Kathy and Phil were strong opponents of the Vietnam War. As a consequence, Kathy and her husband, Ron, immigrated to Canada rather than allow him to be drafted. Ron was a Yale graduate student at the time. Phil, a student at Penn State University, was part of the student activism of the period and radical in his views and activities. In 1972, sorely strained family ties were beginning to ease and be rebuilt. The storm of the late sixties/early seventies was subsiding. It was a hopeful time for Phyllis with regard to her children.

Phyllis' son, Phil, first learned of macrobiotics in the summer of 1969 at Woodstock, New York. At Woodstock, simply prepared whole grains, vegetables, and miso soup were being served to part of the huge crowd gathered there. Phil was intrigued by the mostly vegetarian diet and its potential for helping him feel healthier and improve his concentration. Phil began to practice macrobiotic principles immediately. By winter he unexpectedly found he no longer had asthma. Afflicted with this ailment since childhood, Phil was delighted to discover he could enjoy winter sports for the first time in his life without getting sick. In 1972, when his mother learned she had cancer, Phil was living at home in State College after an absence of a couple years. During those years, while living a hippie lifestyle unapproved of by his parents, Phil attended lectures on macrobiotics given by Michio Kushi in Los Angeles. After getting deeply involved with this study, in 1971 he returned to his home town clean shaven, hair trimmed short, neatly dressed and expressing a respectful attitude towards his parents. Phyllis attributes this welcomed change to the macrobiotic teachings of the Kushis that emphasize respect for one's parents. He continued to share with them what he learned about macrobiotics and traditional Oriental healing methods. When Phyllis received the cancer diagnosis she was just becoming aware of the potential of macrobiotics to heal herself, but she still had doubts about it and about her son. "Macrobiotics was something hippies did," she said.

Two months after the hysterectomy, another biopsy followed. This time Phyllis was told by her doctor she had breast cancer. It was December 31, New Year's Eve. At the insistence of her doctor, New Year's Day, 1973, Phyllis was admitted for emergency surgery. I was given a choice of listening to my physician or this "no good hippie kid." I listened to my physician. I wish, of course, I'd listened to my "no good hippie kid." There was no time to think it out, no time to research the problem as she did before the hysterectomy. The doctor's urgency left her no room to reflect on other options open to her. "The fact I had to go back for a second surgery, the question was where will it strike next? There was a lot of panic, a lot of terror."

Phyllis recalled the trauma of preparing for that operation during a speech she gave at a 1978 macrobiotic conference. "Hospital procedures can range from being ridiculous to terrifying. One of the most terrifying is signing the paper which gives a doctor the right to cut off any part he deems necessary. By the time I was admitted for the mastectomy it was my fourth admission in ten weeks, my fourth signing; and this time I knew what they were going to take. For each operation, there was an initial trip for biopsy, an O.K. from the frozen section, and then a return trip for surgery after more lab work was completed. Another very simple hospital procedure that was sheer horror for me was the presurgical shower. Watching the surgical nurse shave my chest from arm-pit to arm-pit and washing my breasts for what might have been the last time was a very emotional procedure. Before the biopsy, as I washed (and tears flowed almost as fast as the shower) I wondered if I would have none, one or two the next day. I have tried to decide whether the uncertainty or certainty was worse. I honestly don't know." Fear, anger, and a feeling of powerlessness accompanied Phyllis into the operating room that day. These emotions haunted her for months afterwards. The evening following the operation she was in a room by herself. Beside her bed was a large picture window. All she could see was black. Though she was in pain, she would not allow the nurses to give her any pain killers. She knew that whatever they gave her, she would have to get rid of later. She took a minimal amount of drugs.

Amidst the despair and pain she said, "I had this feeling of being drawn out of my bed through the window, out into a black void. I wondered if this was what it was like to die. It was the closest I ever felt to death. That night I was sharply aware that my body and that which I perceived as myself were separate; they were two different things. As I went to sleep I thought I would go out that window and not return. The next morning when I woke, I found I hadn't gone through it. I was in bed. The gratitude for being alive was phenomenal. I thought, 'I made it! I made it! Thank you God for giving me another day!' After this experience, I decided I really wanted to keep me and my body together. And in order to do that I had to do something differently than before. From that time I have tried to create more harmony between the two."

The challenge to do so was immediately at hand the morning she awoke after this experience. "The very first solid food offered me was a bowl of Fruit Loops. When my son saw this he forbade me to eat any of the hospital food. His exact words were, "Mom, if you keep eating that shit, we're never going to get you out of here!"

"Each evening, he would cook for me at home and bring me miso soup, brown rice and bancha tea in thermos jugs." This soup is made with a fermented soybean paste that is used in a similar manner as boullion. Typically, the soup includes wakame (a seaweed) and fresh cut vegetables such as carrots, cabbage, onions and small cubes of tofu (soybean cheese). The soup is garnished with chopped green scallions. In nutritional terms, the soup offers easily digested protein from the soybean paste and tofu; strengthening minerals from seaweed, a surprising amount of vitamin C from cabbage and onions as well as various other nutrients. Widely known for its healing properties, miso soup is eaten daily and given frequently to invalids.

Phil explained, "I started cooking for her and taking soft brown rice with miso soup. I carried it to her for about three days. She healed like people in the hospital had never seen. We brought her home and I kept feeding her. Within a week of her surgery, she went off to New York to get fitted for a prosthesis and the people there could not believe how fast she healed either. Phyllis said the shop attendant who helped fit her examined the smoothness of her skin and was "absolutely astounded" when Phyllis told her it was only ten days from surgery. The surgeon who operated on her was also surprised at her progress.

Allen realized in this short time that eating macrobiotically might give Phyllis a real chance to overcome cancer. He said, "I decided when we brought her home from the hospital that quickly and saw her heal so fast. Phyllis had a history of being a slow healer. A simple burn or cut would take quite a while to heal." About his support of Phyllis' decision not to have radiation and chemotherapy Allen said, "At least with this (macrobiotic) way of eating, if it didn't work you weren't any worse off." About why Phyllis still had doubts about it Allen explained, "I think I accepted macrobiotics before Phyllis because she was educated in science and has a scientific mind. I wasn't. My field is business. Macrobiotics just made sense to me." He was quick to point out though, "Whether I accepted this way of eating was not important. What was important was if she was going to eat macrobiotically, I was going to eat that way too." This was Allen's way of giving total support to whatever Phyllis decided she needed to do to heal herself. About her decision she said, "I was not ready to die. I wanted to live. Modern medicine had done all that it could do for me. For healing, I turned with renewed interest to macrobiotics and to yoga, prayer and meditation. Underlying all this, and a part I can't emphasize enough, was the love and support of my husband, son, daughter and friends."

Support from them was overshadowed, however, by a serious depression for which she had not been forewarned by doctors to expect. In the months immediately following the operations she slipped into a dark well of doubt about herself as a woman . . . fears women commonly are vulnerable to upon loss of breasts and/or uterus. She had questions about herself as a woman and how this would affect her marriage. She wondered what pain or discomfort to expect and the course the cancer might take if it spread. As is normal with the loss of any body part, she grieved. Had she known what to expect she says, "The time may have gone easier for me." She was extremely self-conscious of her appearance. As Phyllis explained, "Losing uterus, ovaries, and breast was difficult as they were fundamental parts of my identity as a woman. Later I had nightmares about imagining them in a garbage can somewhere." She is grateful for the kind response of her family throughout this period, ". . . for tolerating her moods, for the good food they offered and for the love and patience."

Sometimes this was not easy for them to give. The summer following the operation Phyllis went to Canada where the family has maintained a cabin for many years. With daughter, Kathy, a permanent Canadian resident, this also provided opportunity for family visits. About that summer Kathy recalls, "It was awfully hard being around her. I remember she cried for what seemed like the whole summer. She had an awful lot of anger and despair."

Three years later, in 1976, Phyllis had worked through much of the grieving she needed to do and was on her way to restoring order to her life. The threat of cancer was still very real and ever present, however. She was still not confident she would survive cancer. That year, her fears and anger rekindled when articles appeared in magazines and newspapers reporting new research results linking estrogen use to breast and uterine cancer.

The headline of an article in Harrisburg's *Evening News*, August 16, 1976, read: "Estrogen Use May Cause Breast Cancer, Study Says." The study was a joint project of Harvard School of Public Health, the National Cancer Institute and University of Louisville School of Medicine. The report, quoted in the *Evening News*, said: " . . . if a woman on estrogen developed a benign breast tumor, the possibility of breast cancer afterwards was seven times greater than normal. . . ." The article went on to say, "Millions of American women, mostly young and menopausal, regularly take estrogen in the form of birth-control pills." Prior to her cancer diagnosis, Phyllis Crabtree was one of these "millions."

Another article on August 24, 1976, carried a warning from Dr. Carol M. Proudfit (*Journal of the AMA*, August 23) that a number of studies in recent years found increased incidence of cancer in the endometrium, the lining of the uterus, and have associated it with estrogens. This was the specific type of cancer Phyllis had. Then on September 28, 1976, the *Center Daily Times* reported the FDA advising physicians of the following. "Estrogen should not be given to women with breast and uterine cancer. . . ." In 1972, following Phyllis' diagnosis of cancer of the uterine lining and subsequent operation to remove her uterus, fallopian tubes and overies, the doctor prescribed estrogen for her . . . presumably to assist her body's adjustment to "surgical menopause." This operation, as noted earlier, was performed in October. Breast cancer was diagnosed and a mastectomy performed less than two and a half months later. Phyllis could only suspect from this new evidence that her cancers, both of them, could have been medically induced. Intense outrage arose in her when she reflected on this new information, as well as the insensitive manner of the gynecologist who originally diagnosed the uterine cancer.

During this period, when the articles appeared, Phil was no longer living with his parents. The year before in 1975, he had moved to Washington State. Sometime after Phyllis learned about the new research concerning the relationship of estrogen to the kind of cancer she had, Phil made a visit home to see his parents. Speaking of his mother he said, "After the operation, she wasn't much good for a couple of years. She lost her self-confidence. She was alive, but she was scared. Everytime something hurt she was sure her cancer had come back. She was doing the circuit of all the doctors in town. It was hard on everybody." He was confronted with his mother's renewed anger on his trip home. Her anger triggered something in Phil. Describing the occasion he said, "At the end of my visit home, Mom was driving me to the airport. At that time it was up on top of a mountain in the middle of nowhere. As we were driving there, I told her she'd made herself sick and if she wanted to get well, she had to make herself well. All these doctors weren't going to do it for her.

"I'd just gotten fed up with her not being happy, being unhealthy and not enjoying life. I said if she wanted to be healthy and happy it was up to her to do it. And then I hopped on a plane and got out of town."

"I was devastated," said Phyllis. "I sat there at the airport and the tears poured. He told me, 'It's time for you to take responsibility for your own cancer. You are the one who took birth control pills. They didn't force you to take them.' There I was on top of this mountain overwhelmed with feelings. I thought, 'That brash brat!'" Amidst anger and tears, somehow Phyllis managed to get down the winding roads safely and back to State College and her home.

In spite of the upset resulting from the confrontation, both Phil and Phyllis acknowledge this was a turning point for her. Out of the anger generated by Phil's lecture she found new motivation as she began to realize she was the one in charge of her own health. Again at Phil's insistence, she went to a macrobiotic conference on cancer in 1977. There she heard a remarkable lecture by a man who used macrobiotics to recover from cancer. "For the first time," she said, "I felt I was going to live, that cancer wasn't a death sentence."

In a meeting with Michio Kushi, however, he suggested that Phyllis had liver trouble. This information was particularly significant to Phyllis because in her own research she'd found ". . . that women who have endometrial hyperplasia followed by breast cancer . . . the next site would be cancer of the liver." She also had good reason to be respectful of the ancient art of physiognomy or health evaluation based on the observation of external features. In the months preceding the cancer diagnosis for Phyllis' gynecologist, using the physiognomy skills he learned studying macrobiotics, Phil predicted Phyllis was going to have cancer if she didn't change her eating habits. Phil's prediction had a startling accuracy. At the time, Phyllis was caught in a enormous conflict between her respect for modern medicine with its scientific methodologies and what Phil was telling her. She also did not enjoy eating macrobiotically. "It was only something I did because Phil told me I should. Once I got out of the hospital I was about 75 percent macrobiotic in the way I ate and prepared food." However, after her 1977 meeting with Mr. Kushi, she went on a strict macrobiotic diet. "At the conference someone told me in 120 days you change the quality of your blood cells. I said, 'O.K. I'm going to mark it out on the calendar. I am going to eat strictly and if I don't feel better by the time its over, to hell with this whole macrobiotic mess. I'm sick and tired of it.'" Explaining her impatience, Phyllis said, "I am of the generation that was taught to believe science and research can cure any ill — personal, economic or social." Macrobiotics was not based on modern science and research as Phyllis knew it. It was a body of knowledge handed down from teacher to student for generations. The concepts of Ki flow (life force) and yin/yang were totally foreign to her and highly intuitive in their application. In the early forties while pursuing her youthful career ambitions to be a doctor, Phyllis was one of few women who took advanced science courses in college. Her studies included physiology, bacteriology, immunology, anatomy, and histiology, the latter being the study of body tissue. "I had a very technical training, very specific. In organic chemistry, I had to learn to measure things to the decimal point. When you are trained this way you learn that by adding A to B, this will equal C." Macrobiotics challenged everything she was taught. It was not tested out under controlled laboratory circumstances. Explanations as to why macrobiotic principles worked in healing and maintaining health did not make sense to Phyllis within the framework of modern science.

While at the conference, she ate strictly because that was the only kind of food served for the ten or so days of its duration. Growing restless mid-way through the conference, Phyllis quietly ducked out and went to a nearby restaurant for some "good food." "I was fed up and thought of taking the first plane out of Boston." While seated there at the restaurant, however, in came three women. "One was overweight, the other terribly crippled and the third one in a wheelchair. I watched the great difficulty they had to sit down. Seeing this I said 'O.K., God, I got the message. I'll still try this dumb stuff (meaning macrobiotics).' I went back to the conference."

After the conference and while on the way home an amazing realization came to Phyllis. Four years after the mastectomy and prior to the conference Phyllis still had a lot of pain from the mastectomy scar. Women she knew who also had a mastectomy said she would always have that pain. In the plane on the way back from Boston, however, she said, "Suddenly I noticed I did not have pain there and could not believe it." Since then she says she also has found, "All I have to do is eat sugar and that pain comes back."

After she arrived home and ate strictly for the appointed 120 days, Phyllis said, "I felt so much better." Because of several obvious improvements she continued to eat macrobiotically. "I'm a pragmatist. If it works, I'll do it. After the hysterectomy I got a back brace while I was in the hospital because I had terrible back pain. The orthopedic doctor told me I had osteoporosis. A long time urinary problem flared up after surgery also. For the first time since I came out of anesthesia, I felt relief from scar pain. The urinary problem and several other things just gradually went away. I can't remember when I quit wearing the brace the orthopedic doctor prescibed. I was still wearing it in 1977. I just found myself wearing it less and less. I left it in Puerto Rico while on vacation and never bothered to send for it."

Since then Phyllis has returned to Boston several times to see Michio Kushi. In 1979 or 1980 it appeared that she was free of cancer. She also goes every summer to macrobiotic summer conference where she sees a certified counselor. "I consider this my annual checkup. I get information on how things are going, which way I need to go with my diet and what else I may need to do."

Neither of the doctors performing her surgeries said she had recovered from cancer. "One just said, 'You're healed.' The other one commented on how rapidly I healed." Both referred to her incisions. As a precaution she continues to make an annual visit to a gynecologist for a pap smear. "And I have a blood chemistry profile once a year. In 1986, I had a mammogram. I hadn't had one for five years and the doctor was quite adamant I needed one. Also, five years after the surgeries I had a biopsy on the other breast as a result of a mammogram." As for her doctor's attitude toward her experience with macrobiotics, Phyllis says, "Most don't know about it. I just figured there was no point in telling them. When they realize how long I have been without cancer, the comment is, "Aren't you fortunate that we got it all." With a touch of irony in her voice, Phyllis says, "That's the official reaction."

Besides her background in the sciences, Phyllis' reluctance to embrace macrobiotics wholeheartedly is understandable when considering how she was first introduced to it. Phyllis had her first macrobiotic meal in what she calls "a remodeled chicken coop on the other side of town" where son Phil lived at the time. "An enterprising landlord remodeled it. Any wet weather made it smell as though the chickens were still there. Phil was a student at Penn State at the time. The occasion was not too long after he came back from Woodstock where he first heard about macrobiotics. "On a rainy day Phil invited us (she and Allen) over for a macrobiotic dinner. He took it quite seriously when it said, 'Eat whole foods.' He made miso soup, including the onion skins. As a result, we all sat around chewing onion skins. Phil didn't have a pressure cooker so he made his brown rice in a regular pot and it was soggy. I'd never tasted brown rice and, at that point, didn't care if I ever did again. I think he also cooked carrots. The meal did not send me to the corner store eager to start eating macrobiotically."

Phil, nevertheless, was not deterred by his mother's reactions. When he came back from Woodstock he said, "I cleaned the instant breakfast and the other garbage out of my house and sat around quietly starving until my food arrived from New York." By the time his 100 pounds of brown rice and other macrobiotic supplies arrived he'd lost almost twenty pounds. "I went from eating meat and sugar to macrobiotics without any steps in between.

"I was in college in Community Development. I had some pretty radical professors, and in those days they were teaching people to be agents of social change. I enthusiastically worked for peace, organizing communities and feeding people. I was living by myself and thought there had to be cheaper way to eat. I wondered how the rest of the world (i.e. more traditional cultures) ate. I knew they were eating on less money." Describing his own lifestyle at the time, Phil said he also was smoking marijuana and occasionally trying LSD. In terms of food, he added, "I was eating a lot of sugar and had been in a long depression over losing a girlfriend. When I stopped eating sugar and began eating brown rice I started feeling wonderful."

Eventually, he learned to apply correctly the principles of yin and yang to his food intake and way of being in the world. As this transition took effect, the use of drugs ceased to have a place in the new balance he was creating in his life. Within the macrobiotic framework of teachings, for optimum physical and emotional health the goal is to eat foods that are less extreme in energy, but are instead, a balance of the two energies yin and yang. Drugs in any form are considered to be an extreme yin or expansive energy. Their widespread use in today's society reflects an unconcious attempt of the body to balance the extreme yang or contractive energy from heavy consumption of meat. This same principle applies to the excessive and increased use of sugar, an extreme yin, and modern refined table salt, an extreme yang.

Besides being alarmed about Phil's rebellious lifestyle, his parents were concerned he might not be getting adequate nutrition, including calcium, protein, etc. Phil explained to them about the high nutritional content of seaweeds and dark green vegetables. He drove forty five to sixty miles to get organically grown vegetables and persisted to eat the primarily vegetarian macrobiotic diet in spite of their concern. He was pleased and surprised by the results. As mentioned before, since he was three he had asthma. "Every winter I'd go out in the cold and get sick from it. Every May I'd get sick from pollens. I started macrobiotics late summer/early fall. That winter I played outside all winter. I went crazy. I was skiing and sledding and running around. I had so much fun I was beside myself. It was the first winter I could do that without getting sick. I would get up in the morning and feel really awake. I wouldn't fall asleep in class." Inspired by these positive results, he eagerly urged his parents to make the same changes in their eating habits. Phyllis' reaction to macrobiotic philosophy and diet was tempered by consideration of Phil's other involvements at the time. "I just put it all together . . . the student activism, the March on Washington in front of Attorney General Mitchell and macrobiotic eating. They all went with this discontented kid." The fact he overcame asthma made an impression on Phyllis and Allen. However, much of macrobiotics' positive benefits were obscured by Phil's continued involvement in student protests and other activities.

Phyllis' second major encounter with macrobiotics, before the cancer operations, came when Phil invited her to visit him at the study house in Massachusetts. Phyllis accepted his invitation. "My son pleased me by returning to civilization. So I did this to please him." While she was there he made her promise to eat only the food that was prepared and served at the house. To her amazement and welcomed surprise, during the week and a half she was there, she lost ten pounds without even trying. A veteran of many weight loss diets available at the time, weight control was a persistent problem. Her impressions of the visit were mixed. "At the study house we ate at low tables like coffee tables; we had to sit either in *zazen* position or with legs crossed. At that point I was so stiff there was no way I could sit like that so I sat with my feet under the table. Everyone had chopsticks. I still haven't mastered chopsticks and don't see any reason why I should."

In spite of her concerns, Phyllis came back from Wakefield impressed with the ten-pound weight loss. As a result, she began to be more careful about the food she prepared and ate. To eliminate dairy products was out of the question, however. "In junior high school, I once won a prize for writing an essay on why I should drink more milk. I was not about to give up that prize and reduce my milk consumption. The first things we reduced were red meat and sugar. When we cut down on red meat we found we could no longer consume the amount of alcohol we had. So we cut down on that because we could no longer balance it. Then I began reading labels and becoming more careful about prepared foods because that was part of Phil's instructions. It was something that kind of worked its way into our lives. There weren't any real good books out at the time. My first instructions were learned at the study house and from listening to Phil. Cookbooks were hard to find.

"Every month or so something else would happen. Instead of having meat two or three times a day we would have it two or three times a week. If I made a cake I wouldn't ice it . . . little things along the way. I didn't become a serious macrobiotic until after I got sick." Before then she noticed her fingernails stopped splitting, something Phil predicted would happen if she started eating more macrobiotically. It was these little changes like the fingernails and weight loss that made Phyllis begin to think macrobiotics might help her recover. Migraine headaches, from which she suffered regularly, were eased by a massage technique Phil learned in his macrobiotic studies. This also told her there might be something to what Phil was sharing. Allen Crabtree also experienced relief from bursitis and had less indigestion after they made changes in their diet. By the time of Phyllis' operations, both she and Allen we beginning to think there was something of value in macrobiotics. Though skeptical, they each experienced positive changes.

Taking macrobiotics seriously was not easy for Phyllis. For one thing the food did not appeal to her, least of all seaweed. Obtaining organically grown foods required a two-hour drive. Many basic supplies were hard to obtain. The concept of yin and yang as it applied to food and health seemed complex and hard to understand. Many terms and names for foods were Japanese. Along with this in 1977, when Mr. Kushi told Phyllis she was not yet healthy, she said, "He suggested a very conservative diet. Raw fruits and raw vegetables were almost nil. I really missed them and still do though I am not on as conservative a diet. But seaweeds were the worst. I don't have as much trouble with wakame and kombu as I do with hijiki or arame, and I had trouble getting used to brown rice. I never like vegetables. Growing up I only ate vegetables when my mother made me. Part of the difficulty occurs when you go from frozen or canned vegetables to fresh ones; it's a whole new way of cooking and learning not to overcook. One of the things I missed was something crunchy. I crave a chip or cracker. Rice cakes don't do it."

Remembering her transition to eating macrobiotically, Phyllis said, "There is no way I could eat or cook the way I do without Al's encouragement and support." Al, on the other hand, says he had no difficulty with the macrobiotic food. He attributes this to his experience as an athlete in high school when he was placed on strict diets as part of training. "I can remember the coach saying 'No pie, no cake, no candy.' On weekends you can have a little cake or candy but none for the rest of the week — and no smoking. As a wrestler, there were times I had to 'make weight.' I thought I could easily lose six or seven pounds. I discovered it isn't easy, but I got into the discipline of being careful about what I ate.

"Then, Phyllis says the best thing that ever happened to her cooking was my three and a half years in the Army. I was kind of finicky when I was young. The first couple of times they put that mess down in front of me, I said, 'There's no way I can eat that.' Finally you just have to. You'd be out in the field. They'd throw your food into a mess kit and it would be all messed up and you would just eat it. I got used to being able to eat most anything. When we decided to eat macrobiotically I had no problem. There are some things I don't particularly like and there are times when it gets a little monotonous. But I haven't been quite as strict as Phyllis. I eat more like 75 percent to 80 percent macrobiotically. I don't binge on sweets and that stuff. I don't have any desire for them . . . I thought if the diet was going to cure Phyllis, it was certainly going to help me. I figured you can't lose on something that may help you. I thought I'd eat macrobiotically for a couple of years and see how it went. I think its great."

When Phyllis first encountered concepts of Oriental medicine such as Ki flow, acupuncture, shiatsu and physiognomy, it seemed "inane" to her, especially "after having been in a laboratory taking blood samples and working with x-rays. She was, however, intrigued by physiognomy. With this method one can discern the health and well being of a person's internal organs from the external appearance of designated areas of the head, face, ears, hands, feet, and ankles. "The idea of reading people's faces and understanding their health condition fascinated me. I really got into it." In fact, as she learned more about this traditional technique she said, "It provided me with hours of entertainment at airports looking at people who came by and making my own on-the-moment assessments. This ability, however, sometimes places her and Allen, who shares this interest, in awkward situations. "It is difficult to be quiet when we are out with friends and I see dark circles under their eyes. I want to say, 'Do you realize you are in pretty bad shape? You ought to do something about those kidneys.' Or like the friend who came into Allen's store. He had a large bullious nose with pimples on it. Al came in the back of the store and asked Phyllis, 'Do you think we should tell him how bad his condition is?' It was a classic display of a heart problem. Later the man died of a heart attack. He may have been in his fifties."

When Phyllis began to practice macrobiotics, she recalled, "Almost everybody thought we were crazy. It didn't make any sense to them at all. I did not get support from our extended family or close friends. We just didn't talk about it. Mostly it was silence like it didn't exist. One relative sent us steaks for several Christmases after we became avowed macrobiotics. That's one example of the lack of acceptance there was for what we were doing with our lives." Michio says, 'Help the people who are closest to you.' First of all they didn't have the patience and secondly, they wouldn't take the time to do any reading. The whole thing was too ridiculous to consider. The people around me were too stuped in 'The care of your body belongs to your doctor. What do you know about it?' Sometimes I would answer, but over the years I just got quieter and quieter. I have gotten to a point where I don't try to convince." It has been Allen who has enthusiastically told people about Phyllis' recovery and as a consequence many individuals have sought her out. She started teaching a course in macrobiotic cooking twice a year to accommodate them.

Accommodating Allen's and her active life has posed other challenges. One friend told Phyllis, "When I know how you eat I don't dare invite you to dinner." Phyllis gets around this concern by inviting friends to her house. She creates attractive, appealing meals like shrimp and vegetables served over brown rice, a dish similar to Lobster Newburg. As a compromise for her guests, she also sets out a cheese tray. There are simple, elegant desserts she makes from a seaweed based gelatin (agar agar) in combination with fruit juice, a sesame butter sauce and shaved almonds. Tailgating at football games, Phyllis makes a popular, hardy split-pea soup accompanied by other natural snacks made of whole grain breads, vegetables and fruit in season.

Dining out can be a problem, however. Allen says, "It's okay if you go to a high class restaurant. You can get fish and vegetables. But in places like McDonald's, there is nothing we can eat."

When traveling in their camper the Crabtrees say they have a definite advantage eating macrobiotically. "Food does not spoil because we carry dried beans and rice. We use a small pressure cooker for beans, and the refrigerator is big enough for keeping fresh vegetables," explained Allen. On trips to the Caribbean they bring along basic macrobiotic staples and rent accommodations that include cooking facilities. They purchase fresh fish and produce at local markets. This necessity has taken them into areas of towns not normally visited by tourists. Both describe with delight occasions where they bought fish directly off the fishing boats from men who caught them. Phyllis and Allen have enjoyed also discovering what native people eat and local varieties of beans not available in Pennsylvania. Where on the one hand macrobiotics has caused them some awkward moments, it has also opened up a whole new world of adventures and friends. Some of these new friends were met during trips, yoga classes Phyllis regularly attends and the cooking classes she gives through the Center for Well Being in State College. "Going to the Center for my yoga classes I get to know a lot of really fine young people. And I have good friends who are whole generations younger than me. I enjoy that. It's strange, because I identify with them much more than I do people my own age."

In spite of her way of eating, Phyllis always found comfort and solace from friends and members of her church community. Through the difficult years following her surgeries she said she felt a great deal of love, respect, and acceptance from them. "After the surgeries I was so ready to devalue myself because I had less parts on my body than most women have. Especially with the mastectomy, I was terrified to be seen in public. I was so scared everyone would know. The first place I went was to church. This is where I felt at home and felt God's love with these people. That whole church group has been very special."

Working at the day nursery also played an important role in helping Phyllis regain her sense of self worth. As Phyllis explained, "My way of being a Christian was to put it on the line. This is part of why I worked there. Here was a place where my talents could be put to use. One of the things those children needed was love and I had love to give. I felt I had a pretty good in on God's love. After the cancer operations when I needed to be loved back, the day nursery gave it back to me. When I had the feeling, 'Oh my God, am I going to live?' here were these kids who needed me. There was a reason to get out of bed, out of the house and get going."

Phyllis' longstanding love of nature also helped. "After the mastectomy," she said, "I wasn't allowed to drive, but as soon as I was, I would get into the car and drive up into the mountains alone. I would stop the car and just sit." Favorite places were Whipple Dam and Black Mushannon State Park. When Phyllis needed to, she retreated into the still cold of winter where great oak forests cover long high ridges of the Alleghenies. The winter she saw was a sharp contrast of blacks, greys, and white. Armies of trees stood dark and barren against deep snows. From the warmth of her car she looked out at a frozen lake with its broad icy expanse open to the sky. Snow blew across the roads forming soft white drifts in the greyness. Occasionally she saw a deer or other wildlife. Absorbing the beauty she felt closer to God. "I had no memory of praying. Mostly I just sat. I still wasn't very strong. The whole time I was driving on my way there, however, a verse from Psalms came into my mind. 'I will lift up mine eyes unto the hills from whence cometh my strength.' (Psalms 112:1). It was winter and not many people went into the mountains and the parks. The mountains grounded me and were an important part of my healing."

Not too surprisingly, Allen shares Phyllis' love of nature. They both enjoy being outdoors together, hiking or driving to pretty sites in the mountains or countryside. With Allen often beside her, nature nourished Phyllis' spirit in the early days of convalescence.

Two books Phyllis found inspiring and helpful along her road to recovery were *Anatomy of An Illness* by Norman Cousins and *Getting Well Again* by Carl O. Simonton, Stephanie Matthews-Simonton and James Creigton. Commenting on Norman Cousins, Phyllis said, "This was a wonderful book. It's the one where he laughed himself well. That was so many years ago and now people are measuring blood to show when you laugh the quality of the blood actually changes. They are discovering this change can help the body resist infectious invaders. Norman Cousins figured this out on his own. I identified with him. The doctors told him he was going to die. When I had those two diagnoses I was like the kid at a birthday party. I wasn't ready to leave. I wasn't then. I'm not ready now. I don't know when I will be, but I think in fifteen or twenty years I'll be a lot more ready than I am now. It's not that I fear death. There are so many things I still want to do. That's what I felt then. Within a year of when I had the surgery, Kathy adopted a baby. That was my first grandchild and I needed to live to see that child develop. Through my exposure to ideas in Cousins' book, visualization techniques in the Simonton book, transcendental meditation, yoga and my own reflection I became convinced the body and mind have to work together. I've worked on that for a long time. A conference she attended on alternative approaches to cancer in 1979 at Philadelphia emphasized and reinforced this realization. It was at this conference that she first learned about transcendental meditation. "In TM is the idea of getting in touch with oneself. Someone asked me why I didn't use prayer. Well, I used that quite a bit, too. There's a different kind of feeling with prayer. TM is just developed prayer according to practitioners and teachers of it, only here what to do and how to do it are set out for you.

"I got started with yoga in 1979 or 1980. The depression would return and there was fatigue. I drove myself so I wouldn't think. The depression returns on occasion, but nothing like before. One of the messages from yoga is as I get my body stronger, I will clear out my mind." This message dovetailed with something Phyllis learned early in macrobiotics. "Somewhere I remember hearing someone say, 'Macrobiotics is a three-legged stool. One leg is diet. The second leg is exercise and the third is management of stress.' I have worked on all three of those. After the second operation I started to exercise regularly and work on stress reduction." Walking, swimming and yoga all figured prominently in Phyllis' recovery efforts and continuing good health.

Reflecting on the origin of her health problems, Phyllis recalled her dietary history. "I was a perfect set up for cancer. I was born a month prematurely. I was not breast fed." Consequently Phyllis did not receive the extra boost of immunity breast feeding provides. She was frequently sick as a child and because of allergies was unable to wear any fabric other than cotton. Fur collars, orlon, nylon, silk, and blends are a source of great discomfort to her.

"I grew up on the standard American diet. My mother was a Phi Beta Kappa at Syracuse. She read all the current nutrition books and presented us with a well balanced low-cost meal. Mother used to pride herself on her grocery bill being a dollar a day during the Depression, including milk. We had a huge garden and lots of fresh vegetables. It was a status symbol to have lots of meat. I was brought up on a lot of dairy food and my weakness was sweets. Sweets were always given as a reward. It was 'Eat your peas and you can have your cake,' 'Clean you room really well and you can have an extra lollipop,' 'If you are good, then you can have an ice cream cone.' That kind of rewarding has lifetime implications. During college I lived at home. I couldn't eat chocolate or I would get a violent stomachache, and I couldn't eat mayonnaise. In the third grade I had scarlet fever. At sixteen my tonsils were removed and I had an appendectomy.

"As an adult my favorite foods were sweets . . . any dessert. I used to be famous for my chocolate pie, my lemon meringue pie, brownies and chocolate chip cookies. At Christmas time there would be mountains of cookies. Kathy was in Brownies and Phil was in Cub Scouts. If anybody was sick or there was a problem I'd be right there with a chocolate or lemon meringue pie. Recently I went to a neighbor's house whose husband just died. There was partially eaten cake and pecan pie. I don't do that anymore, but a lot do. The idea was 'Sweet is good when you are grieving or sad,' or 'I want to do something nice for you so I'll give you a treat.'"

"I liked meat; in fact, I loved steak. When we got to a place when we could afford it, we had steak every Friday. I used a lot of frozen vegetables. When we had a garden I would freeze my own vegetables and can them. Although macrobiotics emphasizes eating fresh vegetables that are in season, I still do that because I feel they are better than ones shipped from California. As a child I thoroughly disliked vegetables. After I became macrobiotic I realized every vegetable given to me then was overcooked. Now I enjoy vegetables but that was a big switch for me to make. Another thing, my Dad was one of those who insisted you had to clean your plate because of the 'starving Armenians.' I tried hard not to do that to my children."

Another factor in Phyllis' dietary history was her constant attempts to lose weight. She tried "thousands" of weight loss diets. "I used to buy any new diet book that came out. You name it. I'd lose five pounds and then immediately gain it back plus a few more." Phyllis was also subject to constipation and hemorrhoids, a chronic problem. Even after a hemorrhoidectomy she regularly took mineral oil. Among conscientious modern nutritionists, this is known to rob the body of oil-soluble vitamins such as vitamins A, E, and D, essential nutrients for health and functioning of skin, hair, eyesight, muscle tone and the reproductive system. "I used to buy them by the case especially when I could get them on sale. I lugged home quarts of them," said Phyllis. Today, given the quantity of fiber she gets from eating an abundance of whole grains such as brown rice and oatmeal along with beans and lightly cooked fresh vegetables, she no longer has this concern. Variations of beans and rice are mainstays in her diet.

Just as Phyllis' diet and health has been transformed by macrobiotics, so has the kitchen where she used to produce all those cookies, pies, and cakes. In her attractive and efficient kitchen, jars of see-through containers are filled with dried beans, grains, seeds, whole wheat pastas, and seaweeds. Cupboards bulge with neatly ordered cannisters and bottles of foods such as kudzu (a thickener derived from roots), agar agar (a natural seaweed gelatin base), rice vinegar, naturally processed soy sauce, and miso (fermented soy bean paste used in soups). Various herb teas are found there also along with non-caffeine Japanese twig tea, kukicha. Phyllis is proud of her kitchen, a fact that is apparent when she shows it to visitors. It's here in this pleasant work space where she also conducts macrobiotic cooking classes.

Considering the diet she ate while growing up and then as an adult Phyllis made the following observation. "My diet was always very extreme. The understanding of yin and yang helped me understand how it affected my body. Learning this helped me overcome some of my anger at modern medicine and medically induced diseases. In the beginning I had much anger toward the doctor who put me on birth control pills, the same doctor who also put me on estrogen. Understanding it that way (within the framework of macrobiotics) helped. I can control the quality of my blood by what I put into my body and thereby control the possiblity of cancer. I was always a take-charge person. All of a sudden, when I first learned I had cancer, I had no say. I was out on the table and people were carving me up. Macrobiotics gave me some role in my own health."

Looking back at medical expenses paid out for her illness versus macrobiotic expenditures Phyllis concluded "Compared to other people our age who Allen and I know, we spend far less on food and medicine. Except for the annual check up with the gynecologist, I haven't seen our family doctor for a long time. I did go for the cold I had last winter, but I've definitely gone to the doctor less. Of course, when I want to study with Michio I have to fly to Boston, but in terms of food I'm sure we spend half what others do. Because we eat simply and so well, we have almost no medical bills." Macrobiotic-related expenses also include fees for yoga classes and belonging to the swimming club. "One exercise, walking, costs nothing, " she added.

On the medical side of the picture, after the operations when the emotional impact took its toll, there was added expense for counseling with a psychiatrist. Phyllis believes the year following her surgeries would have gone easier for her if the doctors had been more sensitive and realistic in advising what she might experience after having these types of operations. No one informed her of the grieving or identity crisis she might undergo. A different doctor performed each operation. The first one discounted her need for information about her condition. He referred to himself as a "carpenter" and one of the best she could find. The second surgeon responded to her initial alarm about losing one or both breasts by replying, "You weren't planning to use them again were you?" Angered by this cavalier remark, Phyllis felt it showed a complete disregard for her role as a wife and her identity as a woman.

In all, there were four doctors involved in the two operations. This included the orthopedist who prescribed the back brace when she had so much pain after the hysterectomy. The doctors' general lack of sensitivity was also reflected in what Phyllis described as their treating her like a "collection of so many body parts." Speaking of the need to see a psychiatrist she said, "I had to call in a fifth one to help repair the damage done by the first four."

In the long run Phyllis and Allen both consider macrobiotics a very economical way of life. The fact that Phyllis is well and Allen has not gotten sick himself makes expenses associated with practicing macrobiotics worth their investment of time, energy, and money.

When Phyllis' son predicted she was going to have cancer, he warned Allen if he did not change his eating habits also, Allen would have a heart attack. It would be brought on from Allen's having had "too much beef and booze."

"I was a typical World War II veteran," said Allen. "I never drank before I was in the service. When I was in Europe during the war five-gallon cans of wine were strapped on the side of jeeps and tanks because there was no water. During the occupation, every night we all boozed like crazy. After the war I came home and ate meat two and three times a day. In 1972 I weighed 185 pounds, had a pot and was on my way to a heart attack with my friends. Phil said we both had to clean up our act. After Phyllis had her surgeries she opted for no radiation or chemotherapy. When she chose to eat macrobiotically it was no sacrifice for me. I said, 'I want you around. If you are going to eat that way, I'll eat that way.' Others come to Phyllis and their families can't make the change and watch their loved one die.

"Frankly, I like to eat this way because I don't get indigestion. The only way I get indigestion is when I go out and eat what I call 'White man's food' for awhile, and eat a couple of desserts. I like the way I feel eating macrobiotically. I have a fantastic amount of energy. I don't really notice it until I'm around people my age (mid-sixties) and they say they can't do this or that. Their bones ache or there are other things.

"I get an ache and a pain every now and then. I had bursitis in my shoulders about fifteen years ago about the time I started eating this way. If I moved quickly or reached up over my shoulders it would ache. Within several months after I started changing my diet, it went away and I haven't had a problem since.

"I had a large bump on the side of my foot next to the big toe and thought it was bone. I would get a sharp pain across that joint when I stooped for any period of time. That doesn't bother me any more and the bump just went away. I also don't have dandruff anymore. But the main thing is I have a tremendous amount of energy. I just don't get tired. Many of our friends are ten to twenty-five years younger than we are, and I don't have any problem keeping up with them. Most people I know who are my age don't even try to do some of the things I do routinely. If I go up into the mountains to cut wood, they may come along and watch, but very few will pick the stuff up and throw it into the truck. They say 'I'm not about to do that.' Some of the logs I move around are eighty and ninety pounds."

"Most of my buddies who knew I ate this way are dead. I was in a reserve group as Battalion Commander. There were two officers. One was the Executive Officer and the other in charge of training. One had diabetes and died of a heart attack. The other had a first stroke and then three or four years later died of a second stroke. Both ate the way I used to . . . red meat and booze."

The Crabtree family has seen other benefits from eating macrobiotically. During the same time Phil was insistently urging Phyllis and Allen to adopt the macrobiotic way of eating he was also urging his sister, Kathy, to eat this way. Phil explained the reason for doing so. "My sister had been married for eight years. For three years she wanted children, but wasn't able to conceive. One of the times I visited I gave my sister the same dispassionate instructions I gave my mom. I told her the reason she didn't have any babies was because she wasn't healthy. And, if she wanted to get healthy, she would have to do it herself. About that time she and her husband adopted a baby girl. She also started changing her diet and became very interested in natural foods. Within a year of adopting a baby she gave birth to one. Now she has total of four daughters."

Kathy says she thought her brother "was pretty arrogant" considering his own lifestyle at the time. Kathy admits she was angry at Phil, but she began to cook macrobiotically for herself and her husband Ron. Prior to Phil's lecture on macrobiotics, Kathy was using vitamin supplements recommended in Adele Davis' books in an effort to strengthen her reproductive system. "But," she said, "I thought there had to be a better way than taking three hundred pills everyday." That was one reason she gave macrobiotics a try. Kathy also practiced Hatha Yoga, particularly one exercise that massages the internal organs. "I think it was a combination of macrobiotics and yoga that helped." When she became pregnant within a year of starting to cook and eat macrobiotically she said, "That was pretty strong evidence."

"Also," she added "as a result of my cooking differently my husband's hay fever disappeared. Ron used to have a terrible time every spring and fall. He would be almost completely debilitated in bed with a fever and taking five antihistimines a day." As a consequence of the positive results they had from eating this way, both Kathy and Ron became strong advocates for macrobiotics themselves. Commenting about the effects of macrobiotics on her life, Kathy said, "Actually, I ended up being much too fertile. I have four children. Laura's thirteen, Emily is twelve, Heather is eight, and Esther is four. We never planned to have any of them except the one we adopted." On the plus side, however, about her mother she said, "One of the things that helped her get better was having grandchildren and wanting to see them grow up; that gave her a new goal." Phyllis thoroughly enjoys Kathy's large, happy family especially during summer stays at the cottage in Canada when all three generations are together for weeks at a time. Like her mother, Kathy has a special interest in children and is certified to teach kindergarten through sixth grade.

As a result of Phyllis' encounter with cancer and macrobiotics her perspective on life has changed significantly. "The biggest thing that came out of my illness was a feeling of gratitude for just being alive and also a reordering of priorities. Twice I was confronted with the very real fact that I may not live too much longer. I had a lot of convalescent time to consider, 'If I'm not going to live much longer what's important for me to do in the time I have left?' For the last few years I've been working not to be such a perfectionist. I think I've made progress though I do have lapses. I realized part of my illness was due to stress and the source of stress was my drive for perfection. Also, through interest in Eastern medicine, I began to read about Buddhism and different religions along with less conventional approaches to solving problems and eating. This has made me less judgmental. I don't take different behaviors personally. I now wonder what is going on with a person. I think I let go of some friends since my illness and the realignment of my priorities. I decided some things were not worth it. Some people have just gone by the wayside and that includes some of our extended family. The result is much less stress. I don't see the Buddhist influences in Oriental philosophy being in conflict with my Christian beliefs. I don't think I would become a Buddhist, but it has opened up different ways of looking at life. Through my reading and research, if I find an idea in Buddhism that will help me, I don't see that's going to affect my relationship with God at all. I believe God gave me a very good brain. Instead of my saying, 'God, do this or that for me,' my approach is if I have a good brain, I need to go and figure out how other people survived, what they've done to heal themselves. If I find something works in my life I use it. I had a hard time struggling with why God did this to me. In that context I think macrobiotic teachings were more helpful than the biblical. Macrobiotics said, 'God didn't do this to you. You did it to yourself. Look at all that fruit and sugar you ate. Look at all the exercise you didn't take. Don't go shoving this onto God. He gave you a good body and you abused the heck out of it.' Then you read enough and you know God is a loving and gracious god. He doesn't sit up there and say, 'Today you get cancer.' I had to work through all that. After I did, now I feel closer to God. Some people have trouble getting up in the morning. I usually get up at 6:30 A.M. and I'm thrilled to be given the gift of another day."

The teachings in macrobiotics have challenged Phyllis from her first meeting with them. It was like, "You believe this? Forget it. You believe that idea? Forget that." She was forced to reexamine basic beliefs about life. "One statement I'll never forget that Michio made was that 'One needs to be grateful if one has cancer.' If I thought other statements in macrobiotics were ridiculous, that one took the prize. He was right, but at the time I could have thrown the book at him. Of course, now I'm extremely grateful. Having cancer made me stop and ask, 'What are you doing with your life? Who's in charge?' When I realized I wasn't, the cancer made me turn everything completely around. If I had continued along with all those minor illnesses I had for years I'd probably be dead by now. It took something as serious as cancer to make me reexamine my life. In addition, I feel grateful to macrobiotics for my health and Al's and also for bringing Phil back to me. And then we have these granddaughters. They are a living testament to macrobiotics."

Allen also observed changes in his own outlook on life since Phyllis' cancer diagnosis and involvement with cancer. "If anything I'd say I'm more tolerant than I used to be. Since I accepted a whole new diet and found how narrow minded people can be toward that, I think I'm a little better at accepting differences in other people. The whole experience has brought Phyllis and I closer together. I think it's the realization that we are not immortal. Often times as we get older, we begin to take each other for granted. When you have to face the fact one or the other of you is going to die, you don't know when, but you know it's a lot sooner than you thought . . . you begin to say, 'Hey, we'd best be getting along on some things and talking things over as well as going out of our way to enjoy life.'"

Allen says his relationship with his children is also closer. "It's sort of like we are in there against the world. There aren't many people who choose vegetarian-macrobiotic eating. All four of us do. If we didn't there'd be conflict when we got together for dinners and things. That, however, isn't a problem. Also I think I can accept my son's way of life better because of it. I can cite for myself, it was my son that got me interested in this. I might not agree with his lifestyle to some extent, but the fact that Phyllis and I are both healthy and alive we owe to him. When I get ticked off at him, I say to myself, 'If he hasn't done anything else, he's certainly improved the quality of your life and that's not too bad a contribution.'"

For several years Phil has lived in a blue-collar neighborhood in Seattle. A couple of years ago he married and is now the proud parent of a daughter. Over the years, in addition to earlier college work, he has worked as a machinist, studied engineering and physics, been a shade tree mechanic and done odd jobs in construction and surveying. He's grown much of his own food in a front yard garden and enjoys making his own beer and sauerkraut. Presently he does most of the cooking for his family. In the fall he makes cider. Because carpenter ants did serious damage to the structure of his house, he recently tore it down and with his own carpentry skills built a new one on the same lot. His wife, baby and he rented a house across the street until their own house was at a state of construction where they could move back. Phil agrees "urban homesteader" would adequately describe the way he lives his life. He is a generalist in an age of specialists. The radical concepts of social justice to which he was exposed in the Community Development Department at Penn State in combination with the censorship he experienced when he tried to apply these concepts had great impact on who Phil is today. About his activities during the late sixties and early seventies he said, "Everybody taught me you were to like people who weren't your color and be for justice, equality, peace, and freedom. When we got a chance to apply what we learned, people thought we were out of line. At the time I was thinking of the ideals I was raised with and trying to give them a practical application. Frankly, the whole experience ruined me on being middle class."

Phil's wife, a labor and delivery nurse, works half time. At the time of this writing, Phil was still finishing his house. "When my wife goes to work, I take care of the baby. When she is home, I work on the house." During the time the baby was still nursing, Phil would take her to the hospital so his wife could feed her. "We have a nice happy baby because she is not being raised by strangers," Phil said. "It's fun, but it's certainly a lot more activity than I'm used to."

Regarding his persistent efforts to get his parents and sister to practice macrobiotic principles of eating and healing, Phil shared the following. "I haven't been one to get a regular job like others do. I've never been into that. Macrobiotics is something I have done with my time that is positive. At one time in my family I could count five people who were living that wouldn't be if I hadn't been macrobiotic and gotten my family interested in it.

"I take seriously the philosophy of macrobiotics and the Buddhist teaching that you have an obligation to your parents because they enabled you to be on earth. It was useful to me to have the opportunity to repay some of that obligation. It seemed like for Mom it put us on a more equal basis. She had a rough delivery when I was born. And then she a bladder infection that occurred when I was born and lasted until she got into macrobiotics. It seemed to even out the karma to relate to each other as equals. I began to see my parents as people. My having something to give them helped me. They could see me as a person who had something to offer and I could feel I was honoring my father and mother."

Overall, Phyllis feels closer to both her daughter and son for their encouragement and support. Their sharing macrobiotics has been an important part of this support. Thinking about her son's role in her recovery, Phyllis said, "It's very unusual for a son to give birth to a mother which is basically what he did. He gave me a second crack at living. I gave him his opportunity. He gave me my second opportunity. This has developed into a very strong and important relationship. Considering all the trials and tribulations during his student and hippie days, that helped a lot.

"I remember the first step back from our alienation. He told me, 'Michio said I was to thank you for the care you took of me *in utero* (in the womb). By reading my physiognomy he said you did a good job of development when I was *in utero*.' I think that was the first positive thing Phil said to me in five years. We went on with our healing process from there. Back then I hadn't gotten into physiognomy. I think at that time if Phil said anything positive to me I would have been thrilled. I probably didn't question the validity of what he said but the fact that 'Oh, my god, he said something nice.'"

After twenty years as director of the day nursery, Phyllis resigned in 1981 but stayed on as a volunteer driver and taught once a week. In May 1986, when Allen sold his jewelry store, both retired. "That's why it's so important for me to stay well. My kids are grown. My husband's retired. We are fortunate enough to have enough money that if we want to go, we go. No children hold us up. So it's all the more reason to take care of ourselves."

Accordingly, macrobiotics continues to influence Phyllis and Allen's choice and preparation of food. Allen says, "I figure I'll eat this way for the rest of my life."

Phyllis still teaches a six-week macrobiotic cooking course twice a year to twelve to fourteen people at a time and plans to continue doing so. "I finally worked up my courage and started a cooking class. I didn't start one for a long time because I couldn't say the food is delicious like Aveline (Kushi) does when she tastes a dish she's just prepared with seaweed. The reason I finally began to do it is that I was getting so many questions. I was spending an incredible amount of time meeting individuals. I thought if I was going to do this I might as well teach a class on it. People pay for this course, but it goes to the Center for Well-Being. This is a way I can help the Center, and I need the Center because that's where I go for Yoga classes." Phyllis paused for a moment and laughed, "I'm sort of the local macrobiotic guru." In all seriousness, however, she said, "I found the best way to share this information is in the cooking class." Likewise, she encourages everyone who comes to her classes to go to macrobiotic summer camp in order to deepen their understanding of the principles and terms. Phyllis finds this helps. "When you are brought up on the four basic food groups it's confusing to shift to the concept of yin and yang when there are no hard proofs and data in the Western sense."

Laughter comes readily to Phyllis and there is a comfortable affection between her and Allen. "We still have an awful lot of fun together," says Allen. The excitement of their new found freedom after a lifetime of hard work and serious endeavor is apparent and infectious. Both speak with the enthusiasm of children just let out of school for summer vacation as they talk about previous trips and ones they plan to take in the near future. Though it's hard to stay strictly on the macrobiotic diet when they travel, there are strategies they employ to ease the situation. Phyllis says, "When we've gone to the Islands, I made a point to do my own cooking." When cooking facilities are not available, they choose their destination with food requirements in mind. "I'll do very well in Baha where we go to watch the grey whales. There I have a choice of fish. I don't get brown rice, but there will be fish and fresh vegetables. That's one of the reasons we are going back this year." Another reason is the people they met there. "Though they are not macrobiotic they are vegetarian and eat similarly to us." Allen observed, "People who care about being healthy and what they put into their bodies also seem to care about animals and the environment. That's important to us."

When the Crabtrees travel in the camper, Phyllis said, "I load it with beans, rice, miso, soy sauce and all the things I need to cook. Two years ago we went all the way to Arizona. We started out and just went west visiting friends along the way. We stopped at the Grand Canyon and camped there, but there was snow on the camp tables and we decided to rent a room. We had a great time in the Arizona desert. This year we plan to go to Florida. Without macrobiotics, I couldn't even get in and out of the camper, especially if I still had a bad back. It does require planning though. You can't expect to travel all day, stop and expect a meal in a half hour. We took the camper to Nova Scotia a year ago and that was fantastic. On our way home, we stopped at a place in Maine for freshly cooked lobster. It was cooked there on the spot. We had with us some Nova Scotia smoked salmon. It was a beautiful day. We were sitting along a river where we could look across and see Bar Harbor. A sea gull came by, and sea birds in the water scolded us as we ate our lobster. I had made brown rice in our small pressure cooker and cooked vegetables we'd picked up somewhere. It was wonderful."

There are many other trips ahead of Phyllis and Allen, visits to see their children and grandchildren as well as trips to visit old friends and discover new places. Whatever road they travel down on life's long journey one can be sure they are well equipped to appreciate and value every moment of it.

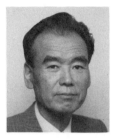

4

Kit Kitatani
Stomach Cancer

There is a unique intensity about Katsuhide Kitatani. He is a man who does not command immediate attention when walking in a room, but has a quiet charisma that one can sense more privately than in a group. It is evident in his eyes, which are soft brown and gentle, yet express intelligence, wisdom and compassion; in his voice, which is clear and calm, yet speaks with authority; and in his gestures, which are simple and direct, yet convey a sense of power and strength.

It was with the same calmness, clarity and strength that Mr. Kitatani took the news eight years ago that he had inoperable cancer of the stomach and there was no cure or hope for his recovery. He accepted the grim news without much emotion or expression, due to his deep religious foundation and profound belief in accepting what life has to offer.

Now, more than seven years later, Mr. Kitatani is still alive, without a trace of cancer in his body. What led to this dramatic recovery is a story that he tells with controlled passion, and with an obvious gratefulness and pleasure in having survived to tell his tale.

Born in Japan in 1935, Kit, as he is called in America, began working for the United Nations in 1962, first in Indonesia, until that country withdrew, and then in Pakistan until 1967. From there he was transferred to New York City, where he stayed until recently moving to Burma. He has traveled all over the world on behalf of the UN as a development specialist, which is similar to an ambassador position, assisting various governments to tap the many resources of countries that were not as yet being utilized. Through this technical assistance, the UN has offered financial assistance as well as technical advice through the United Nations Development Program, or UNDP.

A short, lean and handsome man with straight dark brown hair and angular features, Kit weighed about 177 pounds back in 1983; one of his favorite pastimes was eating, which he did often and copiously. With the ability to travel all over the world, he prided himself on being able to eat in the best restaurants and what he considered to be the finest of cuisines. "Like any other American, I thought I was eating very well. My diet was pretty typical standard American, complete with packaged foods containing preservatives and artificial colorings," he explained. "I grew up hungry during the war, so I became obsessed with feeding myself well. I especially loved anything unusual or exotic. And with my appetite, I thought I had another set of teeth in my stomach." Everywhere he traveled he'd seek out the best restaurants and eat the finest foods he could find. He prided himself on being able to spend any amount of money on food and, as a result of his indulgences, was quite hefty.

Working under intense strain, Kit began having trouble sleeping and was feeling lethargic, as well as more tired and nervous than usual. While visiting Laos and Thailand on business he developed a sore on his tongue, which he thought was the result of some tropical disease or worm he might have picked up from eating exotic food in the Orient. He also noticed his appetite waning, which was alarming, since he usually loved to eat. Thinking his stomach might possibly be the culprit, he started popping pills. Since his doctor recommended that he drop twenty pounds, he started eating apples whenever hungry to reduce his weight and appease his appetite. He found that after a while he did lose weight, but at the same time his energy level and stamina weakened.

Upon returning to New York City, Kit went to a doctor to find the cause of the persistent sore on his tongue, as well as his lowered immunity. A peptic ulcer was diagnosed and pills were prescribed. For three days Kit took the pills, but the problems continued. Still unsure of the cause of Kit's problems, his doctor performed an endoscopy, which required him to swallow, under anesthesia, a hollow tube which would show the condition of the stomach. What the doctor found was not only a huge ulcer, but also something in the middle of the ulcer, which he called a suspicious tumor. A sample of the tumor was sent to a laboratory for a biopsy, but in the meantime, the doctor, who Kit knew was one of the best stomach and colon specialists in the country, recommended immediate surgery to remove the tumor. Three days later, on February 15, Kit had three-quarters of his stomach removed. After the operation the doctor explained to Kit that most of his stomach had to be removed because of cancer, but fortunately the disease hadn't penetrated the stomach wall. Kit knew at the time his condition was serious but was relieved when he heard the doctor's report. "I was an incurable optimist in those days," he remembers. "I didn't immediately connect my operation, or the cancer, to death, as such."

When the doctors first told Kit he needed an operation, they also asked to speak to his wife, Akiko. A detailed discussion followed, none of which was disclosed to Kit. The doctors informed her about the seriousness of her husband's illness. "My wife and two boys, who were freshmen at Columbia University at the time, took the news rather nicely. They weren't upset, or at least they didn't show it in front of me. They were quite composed, quiet and relaxed," Kit said.

With little emotion Kit also accepted the news of his cancerous condition rather matter-of-factly. He felt that what was happening to him was his fate, and just thought it would be best to follow the doctor's orders. He spent the next twelve months recovering in the hospital and began making plans for his work and family life after leaving the hospital. But the worst news was yet to come. A couple of days before the discharge date, Kit was informed of the biopsy results. The cancer apparently had metastasized throughout his lymph system. The prognosis was even more distressing. A tumor could pop up anywhere in his body at the time, possibly within six months time. Privately the doctor told Akiko that her husband had maybe two years left to live.

Now with the news of his doomed condition, an agony of questions and answers whirled around in Kit's mind. He wondered, "If I have this tumor possibly coming back, how long do I have to live? I came to my own conclusion: a year, maybe two. Three at the most. So what do I do in the next three years?" Kit recalled a movie about an old civil servant who also had stomach cancer. With only six months left to live, he was determined and finally succeeded in creating a small children's park in a big city before he died. Now Kit thought about what he wanted to accomplish with his three, maybe less, remaining years. A good friend visited him at the hospital, and after a long philosophical discussion, Kit came to grips with his condition and with a clear mind mapped out his three-year plan. They agreed that he should go back to work in the field, continuing as a resident representative of the UNDF, developing part of the world. "In a way, I didn't agonize over my verdict. It was a psychological thing, and I was feeling all right in this respect. I had a mission. I realized that with this plan I could work to my heart's content at something that was of service, then die peacefully and satisfied, without any pricks of conscience," Kit said.

After his operation Kit was in pain from the incision but had no effects from the cancer in his lymph system. Feeling psychologically satisfied, he returned home to recuperate before beginning chemotherapy. During his home stay, his boss's wife called Akiko one day concerning a program she had seen on television. It showed a doctor being interviewed about a nutritional approach to cancer. Akiko tried to get more information about the program, but none was available. She soon forgot about it.

A short time later Kit's chemotherapy began. It consisted of two shots of medicine daily for five consecutive days, followed by a five-week respite, during which time his white blood cell count was supposed to come back to an acceptable level. Then the same process was to be repeated. The doctors waited the five weeks, but Kit's white blood cell count stayed low. They kept waiting, but after ten weeks the count stayed the same, hovering at a very low level.

At this point the oncologist was very much alarmed and reached the conclusion that Kit had a very peculiar constitution. He said that as a result of the chemotherapy, Kit's bone marrow stopped producing blood, an unusual condition under the circumstances.

Since the doctor was forced to discontinue further treatment of the chemotherapy, he explained to Kit that he had no other form of treatment to offer him and suggested he wait and see what might happen. Since the stomach tumor, which was relatively small, hadn't penetrated the stomach wall, perhaps the cancer wouldn't spread further, he reasoned. But Kit was outraged. "Don't be silly," he retorted. "You can't just drop me like this. Isn't there anything you can do?" The response of the doctor was simply stated. "Nothing. We have to leave it to God."

Upon returning home Kit now had a new set of problems to deal with, which he handled in the same calm reserved way. Again he accepted what was happening to him, whether it meant continued life or an early death. Towards the end of March a very close friend of his was planning to get married and invited him to the reception and cocktail party. Upon arriving at the party, the first person he met was Joyce, an ex-staff member of the UNDP. Kit was surprised to see her, since the last time they met was in December 1982, when she was suffering from lymphoma and going through chemotherapy. "She looked like a ghost then. Her hair was gone, and we thought for sure we would be losing her very shortly," he said. "But at the party she looked radiant. Her hair had grown back and she had rosy cheeks She looked so wonderful. I asked what happened to her."

Joyce explained that she was on macrobiotics. "What sort of economics is that?" Kit asked. He remembered thinking that as an economist, macro meant macroeconomics. Upon further questioning he discovered macrobiotics was a diet and that Joyce was getting stronger and healthier by eating foods like brown rice, vegetables and miso soup. She was following the advice given to her by a macrobiotic friend who also happened to be a cook. "You're kidding?" was Kit's response. "Tell me more about this macrobiotics."

Joyce apparently didn't want to go into details about her new diet but suggested instead that Kit get himself a copy of the book

Recalled By Life by an author whose name she couldn't recall. The following day Kit visited about five book stores in Manhattan until he finally found the book. Dr. Anthony Sattilaro was the same doctor his wife heard was being interviewed on television and had talked about healing cancer through diet.

Kit read the book in one day and came to the conclusion, "If this Italian-American doctor can do it, then I can do it. It worked for him and maybe it will work for me. And besides, it is just like Japanese food. Even though he hated the food at first, he thought, "Since I'm Japanese I know I will love it. So I'm going to give it a try."

Back in the office, Kit asked his colleagues to track down a macrobiotic center in New York similar to the one in Philadelphia described in *Recalled By Life*. None was to be found, although a macrobiotic restaurant, Souen, was discovered. Kit called the restaurant, eager to talk to anyone who could give him information about macrobiotics. A waitress answered the telephone, and a series of questions came firing at her. "She was embarrassed because I was a bit too much for her," Kit laughed. "She put the owner on the phone and he spent quite a lot of time answering my questions. He was very kind to me." In addition to explaining the basics of macrobiotics, the owner directed Kit to a bookstore on Fifth Avenue called East West Books. The following day Kit went there and bought a couple of Michio Kushi's books and several macrobiotic cookbooks.

Kit remembers it was the first of April when he took the books home and announced to his wife that as of that day they were to follow only the recipes included in the cookbooks. "She never questioned or complained to me. She cooperated without hesitation, and for this I really thank her. She also started eating the same way," he said.

Kit began networking with other macrobiotic people and lecturers in New York and beyond. With Akiko, he attended a lecture in New Jersey by Murray Snyder, a senior macrobiotic counselor, and both were impressed with what was said. After the lecture, Murray agreed to meet with Kit. He confirmed that they were on the right track with their initial pursuit of macrobiotics. Murray said he planned to be in New York City in June, so a followup meeting was scheduled. Kit and Akiko returned home and continued with their amended diet.

In June, Murray called to say he had to cancel his trip to New York, but could Kit come to Baltimore instead. Kit decided it was too far and refused the invitation. A day or two later, Joyce, the woman who originally introduced him to macrobiotics, called unexpectedly. She had an interview scheduled with Michio Kushi in Boston the following day and couldn't attend. She wanted to know if Kit wanted to go in her place. Kit felt the timing was too quick for him, but called Michio instead to see about the possiblity of rescheduling the appointment.

On the tenth of June, Kit and Akiko flew to Boston to meet with Michio. An interview ensued, and Michio outlined a dietary and lifestyle program, not only for Kit but for his wife as well. "He turned to my wife after spending ten minutes with me and said, 'Look, you have some problems,' and proceeded to describe all of her current symptoms. She was flabbergasted." After the meeting Michio and Kit talked at length about the United Nations and their favorite topic, world peace. What was planned as a half-hour meeting turned into a three-hour discussion. "We liked each other right away," Kit said.

Kit and Akiko returned home, and for the next seven months followed Michio's advice very carefully. At the end of seven months, Michio said Kit could add a little oil to his diet. "I was very happy about that. My diet was not what I was used to. And as you remember, eating was my pleasure, so even this minor addition was significant for me," Kit explained. Kit and Akiko continued to follow Michio's recommendations, and they both slowly saw signs of improved health.

At the end of the ninth month, Michio told Kit that his health had returned significantly enough to start broadening his diet somewhat. Aveline, Michio's wife, happened to be listening to the conversation and retorted, "Oh no, be careful not to binge!" Kit laughed when she said that, but knew he had planned to stay on the diet anyway. He stayed on a very careful diet for about twelve months altogether, which consisted mostly of brown rice, miso and other soups, seaweeds, beans, bean products, vegetables and other foods.

In the meantime Kit kept seeing his doctor for follow-up visits. Every three months he would go in for a blood test and another endoscopy. This went on for three years, when the doctor finally announced that he was completely cured. He didn't have to come back anymore.

The doctors each had their own version as to the reason Kit survived his cancer. The surgeon said it was because of his surgical skill. The oncologist said that his blood was fine and to just continue doing whatever he was doing. The only problem, he said, was that his cholesterol count was too low. Other than that he couldn't find anything wrong. Kit explaind to the doctors about his diet, and initially they advised him that he would be foolish to follow it. After realizing he was getting better, they told him to continue with what he was doing, but they didn't want to know more about it. They stopped arguing with him because they could see that what he was doing was making him well. Kit advised his oncologist that he should be on this diet too. "He responded to me, 'I know,'" Kit said.

With his health returned, Kit decided to go back to work and chose Burma for a field assignment. He went there in 1986 to head the United Nations mission as a resident representative. Since he believes that the macrobiotic diet and his positive affirmations were responsible for his cure, he decided that his gospel should be spread. He began talking to people about the diet and established a macrobiotic society in the United Nations. The society expanded very rapidly and, by the time he left for Burma, had about 200 members. They were all health-oriented people who became interested in a macrobiotic way of life and diet. In one project nearly one thousand signatures were gathered to petetion the United Nations to serve macrobiotic food in its cafeteria. Monthly Michio or another lecturer would come to talk to the group, which included high and low levels of UN members, according to Kit.

In Burma, Kit still occasionally gives lectures about macrobiotics and explains how to live in a healthy manner. His talks include information about things like why brown rice is healthy and the drawbacks of sugar and dairy products in the diet. When he is faced with any resistance, he says he does not try to brainwash anybody. He just explains various facts and presents the information for people to evaluate and consider. "I don't coerce anyone. If you make a reasonable presentation, people will listen to you. And anyone who is really interested in improving his or her health will come to me for more advice.

"The pace of life is getting quicker and quicker. All around the world people now have access to modern supermarkets and industrially processed foods. At the United Nations we arrange for fertilizers to be shipped, insecticides to be sprayed, and the symptoms of diseases to be eliminated, without addressing their underlying causes. People talk till they're blue in the face but don't seem to take action," according to Kit.

"Converting the people of Burma to brown rice presents a kind of cultural problem," Kit explained. "Brown rice has a negative connotation because it is fed primarily to prisoners and dogs in our country. It is difficult to change their thinking. I am patient, however, and explain the reason why it is good for them, particularly for those who are suffering from some kind of ailment. I arranged with a diplomatic store in Burma, which is run by the government, to sell brown rice to diplomats. So Burmese people are laughing. Now we have two groups of people in Burma who eat brown rice; one is prisoners, the other is diplomats."

Kit believes that charity begins at home, so he offers lectures to his office staff free of charge. He has about eighty people who work under him, and many of them have changed their diets to include brown rice and have cut down on their consumption of dairy and sugary foods. "It is slowly having an impact," he says.

As a personal goal, Kit would eventually like to retire and return to his home in Becket, Massachusetts, near the Kushi Institute, where he plans to establish a retreat for sick people and for those who seek truth. "I want to keep it small. And I want to combine three things — macrobiotics, or a healthy way of eating, spiritual development, and some kind of physical exercise. One of my sons is a Buddhist monk, and I myself have been a monk three times already. We practice meditation. A Buddhist way of meditation will give a kind of theoretical backbone to macrobiotics. And here in the mountains we can provide any kind of exercise you want. You can walk, chop wood, till the ground, swim and much more. I play golf!" Kit laughed. "If you live in a place where the air is clean, and you eat well and meditate and use your body, one is bound to be healthy."

Kit reflects now on his illness and the factors that may have created it. "I was fifteen when World War II ended. We were starving and lost the will to produce. We received sugar from the American GI's. Soon I was crawling around on my hands and knees and developed skin disease, but I didn't associate it with what I was eating at that time." While working at a U.S. Occupation Forces camp, he developed a taste for processed foods, primarily sugary items like ice cream and ketchup.

Kit concluded his story by explaining the virtue of his goals — established when he recovered from cancer through macrobiotics and a positive approach to life. "By establishing a retreat for others, perhaps I can repay the kindness which I enjoyed from macrobiotic people. I would like to make some kind of contribution to humanity. Through a small but individual approach towards health and peace, I hope to help others to contribute towards world peace in this respect."

Of the various foods recommended on a standard macrobiotic diet, and particularly in Kit's case, one is miso, a dark purée made from soybeans, unrefined sea salt and fermented barley or rice. Traditional miso is aged in wooden kegs for a year or more after being inoculated with koji, a special mold that stimulates a fermentation process.

Miso contains living enzymes and facilitates digestion, strengthens the quality of the blood, and provides a nutritious balance of complex carbohydrates, essential oils, protein, vitamins, and minerals. Miso soup has been valued in the Far East for thousands of years for its healthful properties. As a fermented food, it is easily digestible and its combination of soybeans and grains contain all amino acids considered essential foods in the daily diet. The microorganisms in miso help digest and assimilate other foods in the intestines.

Another claim of miso's benefit is that it detoxifies the body from harmful effects of excessive animal foods, sugar or other extreme substances. Following the atomic bombing in 1945, doctors in

Nagasaki singled out miso soup as one of the primary foods responsible for preventing radiation sickness in a large group of survivors.

In 1982, the National Cancer Center Research Institute released findings that showed the results of a twelve-year study of dietary habits, incidences of degenerative disease and mortality rates of 265,000 men and women over forty. The findings showed that those who never ate miso soup had a 43 percent higher death rate from stomach cancer than those who consumed miso daily Those who did not eat miso also had 29 percent more fatal strokes, 3.5 times more deaths resulting from high blood pressure and 19 percent more cancer at all sites in the body. The researchers concluded that "all causes of death were significantly lower in daily ingesters of soybean paste soup."

Another aspect of Kit's diet included fresh vegetables, which comprise 25 to 30 percent of the daily volume of food consumed in a standard macrobiotic diet. Each day's menu in the diet usually includes a balance of root vegetables, ground and stem varieties and leafy greens, prepared by boiling, steaming, sautéing or less often as raw salad or pickles. Vegetables are preferably locally grown and consumed in season.

` Whole grains and vegetables naturally complement each other, and the importance of fresh vegetables has been recognized by almost all modern scientific and medical groups. Their importance in preventing and relieving degenerative diseases is just beginning to command attention. In its report, *Diet, Nutrition and Cancer*, the National Academy of Sciences recommended daily consumption of yellow and orange vegetables, such as carrots and winter squashes and green leafy vegetables, especially cabbage, broccoli, cauliflower and Brussels sprouts, as part of a prudent diet to help prevent cancer. The American Heart Association, the American Diabetes Association and many other organizations have issued guidelines on vegetable consumption that are similar in direction to the macrobiotic diet.

The effects on mind and body of eating different vegetables has long been studied and accepted by traditional Eastern as well as Western medicine. The most common of these purported healing foods are carrots, which alleviate eye and liver conditions; daikon, which facilitates the digestion of whole grains and vegetables and helps eliminate excess water and animal fats from the body; and fresh ginger, which stimulates circulation of blood and other body fluids. Also, the importance of preparing vegetables is vital in macrobiotics, since it affects their energy and nutritional value. Cooking usually brings out the natural flavor and taste of foods, aids digestion, and improves the proportion of nutrients effectively utilized by the body.

Since human blood has a slightly salty composition similar to the ocean, it is important to balance those foods that grow above the ground with those that develop beneath the sea. Sea vegetables, another important aspect of Kit's regime, were a food he was already quite familiar with, being Japanese. Kombu, wakame, hijiki, arame, nori and other sea vegetables in the traditional macrobiotic diet are quite popular in the Far East. While only 5 percent of the macrobiotic diet is comprised of sea vegetables, they are one of the most important foods to help with strengthening the blood, the heart and the circulatory system. Being rich in vitamins and minerals, as well as fiber, they have been long valued for their contribution toward a flexible body and mind. They are reported to have strong anti-bacterial, anti-fungal, anti-viral, and anti-tumoral effects, as well as giving elasticity to arteries, veins, and organ tissues.

Medical researchers at Harvard University reported in 1984 that a diet containing 5 percent kombu significantly delayed the inducement of breast cancer in experimental animals. Japanese women, whose diet normally includes about 5 percent sea vegetables, have from three to nine times less breast cancer incidence than American women, who generally do not eat such foods.

Common sea vegetables have been found to contain a polysaccharide substance called sodium alginate, that selectively binds radioactive strontium and helps eliminate it naturally from the body. In an article in the *Canadian Medical Association Journal*, it was stated: "The evaluation of biological activity of different marine algae is important because of their practical significance in preventing absorption of radioactive products of atomic fission as well as in their use as possible natural decontaminators."

In Kit's case, and for many others on a healing macrobiotic

diet, the brown rice, miso soup, seaweeds and vegetables served as an example of the daily fare recommended for an extended period of time to heal a particular condition or disease. Kit stayed on a careful macrobiotic diet for about twelve months before starting to deviate. This did not mean he went back to his old way of eating, but rather broadened his variety of foods and styles of cooking, still staying within the recommended macrobiotic guidelines.

One of the main problems with his previous diet, Kit later discovered, was the use of polished white rice rather than whole brown rice as a main food. This practice is common today throughout Asia. Compared to whole grains, refined or polished grains or grain products such as white rice and white flour are deficient in the natural balance of nutrients. Various types of fiber, amino acids, minerals, vitamins, and enzymes are naturally present in the outer layers of whole grains. Almost all of these outer layers are removed in the refining process. Although complex carbohydrates and a small percentage of these nutrients may remain, eating polished grains produces imbalance in the body that contributes to a wide variety of conditions. And, when the grains have been heavily chemicalized, as they are in modern artificial methods of rice production, eating them can contribute to disorders such as stomach ulcers and cancer.

Refinement and polishing of grains became popular in the late nineteenth century and spread throughout the world in the early twentieth century, along with the spread of industrialization. During this time, many deficiency diseases appeared, including well known incidences of beriberi in Japan and other Asian countries resulting from lack of B-vitamins in white rice.

With the spread of degenerative diseases throughout the world, the protective effect of whole grains has started to gain greater recognition. Scientific studies have shown that whole grains strengthen the heart and circulatory system and reduce the risk of heart attack, stroke, and high blood pressure. Epidemiologist Jeremiah Stamler, M.D., an international authority on heart disease, commented, "People subsisting on cereal-root diets have low levels of serum cholesterol and little atherosclerotic coronary disease (clinical or morphological). This correlation has been consistently observed in every (traditional society studied) to date." In an editorial, "Sensible Eating," the *British Medical Journal* concluded, "Few nutritionists now dispute that Western man (and woman) eats too much meat, too much animal fat and dairy products, too much refined carbohydrate, and too little dietary fiber.

"Epidemiology studies of heart disease suggest that at least some of the deaths in middle-aged people from myocardial infarction (heart attack) could be cut by a move toward a more prudent diet — which means more cereals and vegetables and less meat and fat."

At the same time, many nutritional studies show that as part of a balanced diet, whole grains reduce the risk of many forms of cancer. The U.S. Senate Select Committee's report *Dietary Goals for the United States* (1977), the National Academy of Science's reports *Diet, Nutrition and Cancer* (1982) and *Diet and Health* (1989), the U.S. Surgeon General's Report on *Diet and Health* (1988), and the dietary guidelines of the American Cancer Society all call for substantial increases in the daily consumption of whole grains such as brown rice, millet, barley, oats, and whole wheat.

From reading Michio Kushi's book, *The Cancer-Prevention Diet* (St. Martin's Press, 1983), Kit discovered that the modern Japanese diet high in chemicalized white rice, sugar, MSG and other additives probably played a role in the development of his illness and in the high rates of stomach cancer in Japan. Mr. Kushi cited a 1963 study comparing incidence rates of common cancers among people in America and Japan to illustrate how dietary patterns influence the development of cancer. In the study, it was discovered that Americans developed over twice as many breast cancers and over three times as many colon cancers as the Japanese — yet the Japanese were suffering with more than six times as many cases of stomach cancer. As Mr. Kushi explained, these differences were due to the differences in diet between the two countries. Americans consume a larger volume of meat, eggs, cheese, and other dairy products that contain cholesterol and saturated fat. When eaten excessively, these substances tend to accumulate in the lower parts of the body, for example in the colon, rectum, and prostate gland, where they can eventually lead to cell changes that produce cancer. On the other hand, the white rice, sugar, and chemicals eaten in the modern

Japanese diet tend to cause trouble in more upward regions of the digestive system and body as a whole, including the stomach and esophagus. The habit of not chewing well, which is common among modern Japanese and other white rice eaters, contributes to this tendency. When we chew thoroughly, food is mixed with saliva, an alkaline substance that neutralizes the acid secretions of the stomach wall. By not chewing, there is a greater possibility of developing an over-acid condition in the stomach, leading to eventual irritation of the stomach lining and to stomach ulcers and cancer.

When the differences in cancer incidence between the United States and Japan were first discovered, some researchers thought they were due to genetic differences. However, other evidence disproved this theory, especially data showing how the incidence of cancer in Japan has changed over the last forty years, as well as data showing that, over time, Japanese who move to the United States develop cancer incidence patterns similar to those of Americans. Both of these discoveries point to an important role for diet in the development of cancer.

Between 1947 and 1974, for example, milk consumption in Japan rose twenty-three times; egg consumption increased thirteen times. Meat and other popular American foods have become much more common, and the Japanese diet as a whole has changed rapidly in imitation of the West. During that time, stomach cancer has been reduced by one-third — but colon and breast cancer have risen sharply to approach American rates. A primary cause of these changes, Mr. Kushi explained, was the large-scale adoption of foods such as meat, cheese, and other dairy products that occurred following the Second World War. A similar situation occurs with Japanese immigrants to America; after three generations of the new environment and new dietary habits, the rates for colon and stomach cancer automatically adjust to conform to the American standards. In Mr. Kushi's book, Kit also discovered that epidemiological studies from around the world have pointed to a similar role for diet in the development of certain cancers, and that as a result of accumulating evidence, leading public health organizations have issued dietary guidelines for the prevention of cancer. He was surprised to discover that the macrobiotic diet is totally consistent with these preventive dietary guidelines.

Kit and his wife, Akiko, have two sons, Jun and Ken, who are in their mid-twenties and fraternal twins. At the time their father became ill, Jun and Ken were biochemistry students at Columbia University. Upon hearing the news about their father's illness, they reacted with much surprise, especially since he never got sick or had any symptoms of disease until then. In fact, they rarely remembered him even complaining about having a cold or headache. In recalling this experience, Jun said that being Buddhist, they accepted things calmly and peacefully.

Jun remembered feeling very sad at seeing his father in the hospital with such a serious disease. He had lost a lot of weight and looked tired, but other than that had no noticeable symptoms.

In school, Jun and Ken ate the typical American diet provided for them. It included plenty of meat, dairy foods and sugary foods. Being relatively healthy, neither of them thought much about what they ate. And although they ate a standard Japanese diet prior to going to college, which included white rice, they added American foods to their regime when they arrived in this country.

When they first heard about their father's new diet, Ken and Jun were skeptical. In fact, they didn't encourage him to continue. It was only after a few months, when they saw his condition improving, that they began to take an interest. When it became evident that the diet might be the factor that was saving their father's life, they started reading and researching macrobiotics. Jun said it made such common sense to them that they started eating that way too. They began to replace the school foods with what they cooked in their dorm rooms. And while the diet wasn't a drastic change from the way they used to eat in Japan, Jun noticed a feeling of being cleaner than he had ever experienced. Mentally and emotionally he began to feel more stable, and said he began feeling really good most of the time. Once ingrained in the diet, Jun and Ken never considered switching back to their old eating habits.

Another factor that led Jun and Ken into pursuing macrobiotics was seeing the change in their mother. Jun said she is a petite woman with a strong character and a strong will. He said she was typical of most Japanese women — never showing her emotions and maintaining a positive attitude. They saw her becoming much healthier as a result of the diet. She was calmer and happier, according to Jun, and was extremely supportive of her husband by cooking for him without deviating from the diet herself. Jun remembers her saying that she knew Kit would survive his illness even when the doctors said he might not live.

Jun said that he and his family are very grateful for Michio Kushi's guidance and respect his commitment to teaching and spreading macrobiotics throughout the world. Because of Mr. Kushi's infuence, Jun said he has been able to broaden his perspective. Growing up in America with a standard education, he is reminded how Mr. Kushi brought traditional Eastern thinking, philosophy, science and medicine to his family's life. "Mr. Kushi epitomizes the Eastern mind and thinking, and macrobiotics gives us a broad comprehensive way of observing the world and society through history and science. As a result we have become more flexible and open minded. The diet helped eliminate toxins in our bodies, and as a result our minds are fresher, our bodies lighter and we are more flexible, open-minded and have a positive, refreshing attitude," Jun concluded.

In talking with Michio and Aveline about Kit, Michio recalled seeing Kit four times during the course of his illness. Even though the doctors gave Kit a one-year prognosis, Michio felt that through a balanced macrobiotic diet, Kit could reverse the effects of his illness and get well again.

Michio said that Kit's problems stemmed from eating gourmet foods and not chewing well. He said that the biggest problem for most people is their hurry in eating a meal and not taking the time to chew each mouthful carefully.

After following the macrobiotic dietary suggestions, Kit began to get his appetite back, which Michio said was a sign of his healing. After eating macrobioticaly for nine months, Michio said he had improved enough to start widening his diet somewhat. He mentioned that Aveline had been right in suggesting that Kit not deviate from the diet at the beginning. Her observation had been that many people start broadening too much away from a macrobiotic diet, sometimes before their body is ready. She suggested he wait until it was more certain that the cancer was gone from his body until eating other foods. Michio agreed. He said it takes seven years for cells to change, and time is needed for the body to heal, especially in the case of cancer. Michio emphasized that one of the key problems affecting the health of adults today is poor dietary habits as children. Many children are fed infant formulas as opposed to being breast fed. While the data is not conclusive, he mentioned observing a natural strength of immunity in people who were breast fed as children. He said that in the 1940s and 1950s, infant formula was highly recommended for children. It wasn't until the 1970s that breast feeding again became popular. In Kit's case, the fact that he was breast fed as an infant gave him a better chance to recover from his illness. Degenerative diseases don't come on at once, he said. They take years to develop, so often people are doing destructive things to their bodies without being aware of it.

Michio stated that Kit and others who have recovered from serious illnesses through macrobiotics haven't just found a temporary approach; they have discovered what has become for them a basic fundamental way of eating and living. Those who understood the healing aspects of food and diet, like Kit and Akiko, often wish to share this knowledge with others. For Kit this outlet came through his work in founding the International Macrobiotic Society of the United Nations in various parts of the world, including New York, Bangkok, and Burma.

According to Michio, the natural foods movement started twenty-five years ago with macrobiotics. He said that from the beginning, people began to develop an interest in diet, and different approaches including diets that are low in fat and cholesterol and high in fiber and complex carbohydrates become popular. He mentioned that macrobiotics is spread from person to person and family to family. When once success is achieved, it sparks the interest of others who also desire health and happiness. In this way, personal experiences, such as those of Katsuhide Kitatani and the others in this book, can lead to a healthy and peaceful world.

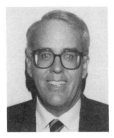

5

Doug Blampied
Leukemia

This is the story about a man who, nine years ago, was told he had cancer and only six months to live. Life for this man had been driven by an underlying need for success in everything he did. He packed in the day with work, overtime, meetings and socials. He ran, sailed, skied and played golf as hard as he worked. He took people and life for granted — going from meeting to meeting, function to function, day to day, with little time left for his wife and family. He never realized that what he was really looking for in life was something he already had.

It is the story of how a man nearly died of cancer, but through a combination of a macrobiotic diet, positive thinking, prayer, a strong will and support from his family and friends, conquered his illness and now lives a life that is quite different from the one he used to lead.

The man is Doug Blampied. Nine years ago, at forty-six, he weighed 160 pounds and was handsome, healthy, and as he put it, "beefy but fit." With his clean cut, good looks and professional appearance, Doug could easily have passed for a vice president, which was a goal he endlessly pursued. As a director of Human Resources for Chubb Life America, a New Hampshire-based insurance company, he was consumed with his job of overseeing a staff of twenty-three located in four areas of the country. He was with the company eighteen years, starting as a manager of accounting when there were only 150 employees. His current position entails hiring and firing personnel, handling policies, procedures and benefits payroll for a staff of 1,500.

The summer of 1982 was a typical one for Doug with a full business and social calendar, although he was more tired than usual. The end of summer plans were capped off with a sailing trip around the islands of Nantucket and Martha's Vineyard with his wife, Nancy, and another couple. The trip was enjoyable for Doug and he felt rested and refreshed. When he returned home, however, he couldn't quite get back his energy level. Coming down with what he thought was a flu or virus, he went on with work as usual. But his fever wouldn't go down, so he finally decided to see his local physician. After a routine check, he got dressed and returned home to bed.

Six hours later, the phone rang. It was the doctor's office with an urgent message — get to the hospital immediately! With questions and fears racing through their minds, Doug and Nancy hurriedly packed and headed for the hospital. After checking in, Doug was assigned a room and administered a battery of tests, including a painful bone marrow extraction from the hip.

That afternoon, Nancy sat by Doug's bed as they waited in dreaded anticipation for the test results. The room was shared; a man in the bed next to Doug's was with some visitors at the time. The doctor arrived wearing a serious expression on his face that echoed the sterile white of his coat. Without bothering to pull the curtain between the beds, he coolly made a statement that was to change the course of Doug's life forever. "Mr. Blampied," he said, "you have an acute case of myelogenous leukemia. You need to decide today whether you want to be treated in Boston or at Mary Hitchcock Hospital, and we need to send you there in the morning."

Doug and Nancy looked at each other in disbelief. After a moment of shocked silence, Doug turned to the doctor and frantically pleaded with him, "Isn't it possible you have the wrong guy? Can't we do the tests over again? Could there be a mistake?"

The next morning Doug and Nancy were in Mary Hitchcock Hospital, a teaching facility located in Hanover, New Hampshire. They had chosen Hanover primarily because of the distance to Boston and difficulty parking there. That afternoon more tests were administered and the results were devastating. They confirmed cancer of the blood and also showed cancer in the spinal fluid.

For one of the few times in his life, Doug found himself crying. The thought of an early death was something he hadn't considered since his grandparents and great-grandparents had lived well into their eighties. And even though his mother had died of throat cancer, Doug attributed it to her poor diet and alcoholism. Now the questions were abounding. "What's going to happen to me? What do I do now? How serious is this?" Not only was the thought of death very frightening, he also realized that he wasn't finished with living yet.

Memories of his children flooded through him as he realized he might not see them finish college or get married. He looked with blurred vision at his wife and thought about how little time he had spent with her during their marriage. As he thought more and more, he realized that he had taken people and life for granted — living from day to day without appreciating much of anything. He'd look forward to the weekends during the week, and when the weekend arrived, would be thinking about the following weekend. While he enjoyed many activities, he didn't relish any experience, only the thought of what the next experience might bring.

Family and friends reacted in shock to the news about Doug. He had been known for his vitality, intensity, good health and humor. It was hard for them to believe it was the same Doug they were hearing about.

After getting the test results back, the doctors had to wait for ten days to treat Doug's cancer because he had a high fever. They were afraid he was too weak to withstand the chemicals necessary to halt the spreading cancer cells. As he floated in and out of consciousness, they tried in vain to control the raging fever. Finally, after having little success, Doug's doctor announced, "We've got to get at that cancer," and Doug was prepared for treatment.

The first step was to implant a plastic Hickman catheter into a vein leading to Doug's heart. The tube allowed medicine to be administered and blood to be withdrawn without having to continually put needles into his body.

The fever finally dissipated, but for the next one and one-half months Doug fought the cancer as the drugs were pumped into his body day and night. Life had become unbelievably miserable. As a result of the chemicals, he would wake up nauseated, try to eat, and vomit almost daily, sometimes as many as five times a day. He forced himself out of the bed to bathe and use the bathroom, only to fall back to bed sick and exhausted. Daily the doctor would arrive with a group of student doctors and they would surround Doug's bed and discuss his treatments and examine the various sores on his body caused by chemotherapy. "I didn't mind the students," Doug remembers. "I kind of liked being the center of attention."

With his hair gone and his weight down to 140 pounds, Doug looked like a shell of his former self. He was listless and weak and unable to do much except eat, sleep and get out of bed once a day with assistance. Nancy found herself on "automatic pilot" from the day her husband was diagnosed. She called the superintendent at the school where she taught learning disabled children and received encouraging support as she announced her need to take an extended leave of absence.

Then Nancy began the tedious job of managing her husband's illness. "She was a 'Rock of Gibraltar,' for me," Doug fondly recalls. "She literally moved in with me at the hospital. She ate there, slept in a cot beside my bed and questioned everything the doctors gave or did to me." While totally at the mercy of the doctors and hospital, Doug found Nancy's inquiries and attention to details gave them some control of the situation and a say in the way his life was being handled.

Doug's children offered their support to him, even though he knew it was difficult for them to see their father wasting away. His daughters, Deborah, sixteen at the time, and Jennifer, eight, were regulars at the hospital on weekends. They entertained their father and cheered him up with their visits. On occasion Nancy would bundle her husband up with blankets, and with about five intravenous lines dangling from the wheelchair into his body, roll him out into the autumn chill, just to get a change from the hospital scenery. Doug particularly remembers his daughter Jennifer doing cartwheels on the lawn across from the hospital to cheer him up, as he sat immobilized in his chair. Doug thinks it was the hardest for his son to handle his illness. David, nineteen and a freshman in college at the time, would come home from school once a week to see his father. Doug could see the struggle going on in his face as the doctors continually warned the family about the slim chances for their father's recovery.

Several times Doug's condition became so tenuous that the doctors told Nancy she should make preparations for his death. She made sure the family finances were in order and began making mental preparations for losing him. Doug, however, had other plans. "Even though I felt unbelievably horrible, I didn't succumb to the idea of quitting. I had too much to do and wasn't finished with living yet. From the moment they announced the severity of my illness, I became determined to be a winner and not a loser in the battle. I would look at my wife and children and know that I hadn't done all the things with them I wanted to do. I wanted to live more than anything, and even though the odds were against me, I made up my mind to overcome this illness whatever it took." Statistics at that time showed that most men of Doug's age didn't survive acute myelogenous leukemia for very long.

With the foundation of a strong will, support from family and friends and a determination to live, Doug's recovery process began. While in the hospital, he received daily calls, gifts and letters of encouragement. Over 300 fellow workers signed a 3' x 4' get-well card and had it delivered to his hospital room. "I really felt good about that. It cheered me up," Doug recalls. His boss assured him his job would be waiting when he returned to work and to take as much time as necessary to get well. He fondly remembers the support of doctors and nurses during his hospital stay. "One nurse, in particular, was such a great help to me. One night I was having a really bad night. She held my hand most of the night while I cried."

After a month and a half in the hospital, Doug began to show signs of recovery and was sent home, bald and still very sick and weak. He was taken off chemotherapy and put on a protocol program. As a teaching hospital, Mary Hitchcock often used this type of experimental process to gather data for teaching purposes. It involved selection of a random treatment from a number available for Doug's type of illness. Since none of the treatments was yet proven successful, he became a "guinea pig" for the hospital to determine the success or failure of the method. Based on the results, doctors could decide which treatments worked and which ones didn't.

The plan was for Doug to receive medicine for nine months, consisting of a shot every day for five consecutive days. Then, following a three-week respite, he would continue to receive shots for another five days and so on. With the Hickman catheter left in place, Nancy was trained to administer medicine through the tube leading to his heart. On the third day at home, Doug went downstairs to make himself breakfast. As he sat in front of the television, he noticed something on the floor. He bent down to pick it up and realized, in horror, that it was his catheter; it had apparently popped out of the hole in his chest. He was rushed to the hospital with Nancy applying pressure on the hole for fear he would bleed internally. Fortunately, the area had cauterized, the doctors told him, and they decided against operating to replace the tube.

Without the catheter available, Nancy had to learn to administer shots into Doug's leg. The drugs played havoc with his health, creating a perpetual sickness or fever. "It was like being on a roller coaster," Doug explained. "I'd get shots for five days, then get a fever, have to go to the hospital to recover for four or five days, then I'd have a couple of weeks to recuperate until the next series of shots, and then the same process would repeat itself. The chemicals I was receiving were designed to kill the leukemia cells, but it seemed like they killed a lot of other things besides." Due to the intensity of his fevers, the doctors were forced to halt the treatment after eight months.

In January 1983, Doug decided in order to keep himself busy, he would return to work. At first he'd stay only an hour or two, then go home exhausted. As he got stronger, his time at the office increased to a half day, but unfortunately the fevers caused by the protocol treatments forced him to cut his work schedule short. Most people at the office were friendly and supportive, but occasionally Doug would scare someone away with the story of his illness. He remembers one social function where an associate approached him and asked where he'd been for so long. As Doug began explaining what it was like to have leukemia, the man looked at him with a blank stare, put his drink down and walked away. "I guess he thought whatever I had was pretty contagious," Doug laughed. "Many people are afraid of what they don't understand."

Life over the next couple of months was slow but steady for Doug. He went into the hospital monthly for a checkup, and the tests continued to show his cancer in remission. This meant that less than 25 percent of his cells were leukemic. If the percentage were to get higher, he would need to return to the hospital and continue with chemotherapy treatments.

In April, Doug's doctor decided to do a bone marrow harvest on him. At that time only a few hospitals in the country performed this kind of operation. The first step in the procedure consisted of an extraction of two quarts of bone marrow from Doug's spine. To get the marrow, a hole was drilled into the bone and an instrument with a hook on the end was inserted in to pull it out. Then the marrow was treated with antibodies, frozen and stored, available to be administered back into Doug's body should the leukemia come back. Usually the bone marrow is taken from a donor with matching blood, but in Doug's case, no match was available, so his own was used. A team of doctors arrived from John Hopkins University to perform the six-hour procedure and train the doctors at Mary Hitchcock. Doug was the first patient at that hospital to have the procedure.

At the time of Doug's bout with leukemia, it was rare for a patient to survive a second remission for longer than six months. This meant that if a patient developed cancer a second time, after having a first remission, the chances for survival were slim. In Doug's case, if the remission was lost, the doctors planned to do a series of chemical and radiation treatments to kill the cells around the cancer. Then the stored bone marrow, treated with antibodies, would be replaced into his body as medication. As Doug explained, the bone marrow harvest was a form of insurance available should the cancer return.

When he was released from the hospital, Doug began reading and studying as much as he could about his type of cancer and ways of treating it. He attended a cancer support group and met regularly with fellow sufferers to air his frustrations and problems. He also discovered a pastoral counselor in Concord, New Hampshire, who recommended Carl Simonton's method of visualization. Doug went once a week for counseling and while at home, listened to a tape several times a day that had been prepared by the counselor. The tape, which lasted about a half hour, was designed to help him relax and focus on healing. When relaxed, Doug envisioned the cancer cells as little amoebas or villains in his blood, and then would see Pac-Men swimming up his bloodstream gobbling up the amoebas. Along with this visualization, he pictured the cancer cells leaving his body every time he voided, sweat or blew his nose.

In June, Doug went in for his monthly checkup. He expected the usual clear results and casually dressed to go home. When the doctor came in the room, Doug knew by the look on his face that something was wrong. His cancer count was rising again, he was told, and some other kind of treatment was necessary. Doug was devasted. He assumed that the visualizations and intensity of his healing approach was working. "This really did me in. I was so directed at curing myself and thought I was doing that," he said.

The doctor recommended a bone marrow transplant using the frozen marrow extracted from Doug. He advised against more chemotherapy since Doug's body was already in a weakened condition. He reasoned with Doug, "If we go back to chemotherapy, you've probably only got six months to live after that, so what good would that be? So let's try this new thing."

Doug and Nancy knew that the prognosis was not good. With a six-month life sentence available doing chemotherapy, this left the bone marrow transplant to treat his cancer. Nancy began calling all over the country to find out more about this kind of treatment. Her findings were not encouraging. Of the fifty or so patients treated with this procedure at John Hopkin's University, only three or four were still alive. With little hope from either treatment, Doug and Nancy agonized over their decision. After much deliberation, they finally decided to forego the doctor's recommendations. Doug's strong will again became evident as he reasoned, "If I'm going to live for only six months after treatment with chemotherapy, then I'd rather die without it and die happy. I was miserable during the time I was receiving the medication, and I'd rather live life normally, even if it is a shortened life."

At a support group meeting during this time, Doug picked up a copy of Anthony Sattilaro's book *Recalled By Life.* Doug read with intense interest about the man who had recovered from terminal cancer by eating macrobiotic foods. With his curiosity piqued, he made an appointment at the Kushi Institute in Boston. Although he had read about many other adjunctive approaches to sickness — from colonic irrigations to laetrile — he understood that the macrobiotic approach was non-intrusive and non-threatening. And fortunately, the headquarters were convenient to his home.

Nevertheless, there were doubts. On the way to Boston, he pulled the car over four times to reconsider his appointment. He wondered aloud to Nancy, "You know I don't know anything about macrobiotics except what I read in Sattilaro's book. What if it's a hoax? Do we want to spend the money to do this?" Doug's curiosity got the best of him and they continued.

At the Kushi Institute, Doug and Nancy met with John Mann, who was positive, upbeat and offered hope for Doug's recovery. John gathered a lengthy background on Doug and outlined a dietary program which he encouraged him to follow as closely as possible. With his new diet in hand, and a positive glimmer of hope, Doug took Nancy out for their first macrobiotic meal. "It was just awful," Doug complained. It was "bland, boring and unappetizing. And the seaweed is the worst part." That evening Michio Kushi was scheduled to give a talk up the street from the Institute, and Doug and Nancy decided to stay overnight in Boston to hear him. At the lecture, Doug's impressions were of everyone in the audience listening intently to this man who he could barely understand. He figured he must have something important to say, though, since so many people were listening intently. What inspired Doug most about the evening, however, wasn't what was being said at the podium, but what was being said directly to him.

A man in his late twenties happened into conversation with

him, and to his surprise, Doug found that he had been sick most of his life and had leukemia since childhood. It wasn't until he started practicing macrobiotics that he finally began to feel and look better and eventually became free from cancer. Doug was more than impressed. That meeting had such a profound impact on him that he decided right then and there to start practicing macrobiotics.

Upon returning home, the Blampieds made some radical changes in their diet and lifestyle. "We decided to go for it," Nancy said. "We replaced the electric stove with a gas one, cleaned out the cupboards of foods that weren't supposed to be good for Doug, and supplied ourselves with a complete macrobiotic kitchen." Doug had no problem making the necessary changes. "Hey, if Michio Kushi says cooking with electricity is going to interfere with my recovery, then out with the stove! It was that simple. Fortunately, I had the finances and it wasn't really a problem for me."

Doug and Nancy returned to Boston a short time later to attend a Way of Life Seminar, a two-day intensive program that introduces the basic macrobiotic principles. Upon returning home they discovered a group of macrobiotic friends in New Hampshire who offered cooking classes. "We became very active with that group. We got interested in philosophy and met regularly to share potluck suppers and talk," Doug said. He found cooking classes to be the best way to learn more about the food and to learn creative ways to prepare macrobiotic dishes. "I actually began to enjoy eating the food after learning how to cook it," he said. During this time, Doug also continued with his visualizations, while gradually incorporating other positive changes in his life.

A short time later the Blampieds found a macrobiotic cook who was willing to exchange her cooking skills for room and board. Doug found her to be of great help in making the change to the macrobiotic diet. While there for five months, she made a variety of appetizing dishes. "She had a gift for putting something together seemingly out of nothing, and she knew how to balance and season it so it really tasted good," Doug said. Along with teaching Doug and Nancy how to cook, she showed them how creative and good tasting the foods could be and how to balance the foods in a way that could support their health. For Christmas she made a gift she called "Doug's cookbook." It was a handmade book to be used to hold his favorite macrobiotic recipes.

With his cancer in remission, and feeling better than he had in a long time, Doug thought he had things under control. But the doctor wasn't satisfied. "He advised me to go through another bone marrow harvest just in case, heaven forbid, the cancer should return," Doug explained. While his first harvest was still being saved, the technology had improved significantly since that time, so the treatment had even more chances of success. Doug and Nancy learned that the doctor at Mary Hitchcock who worked with this form of treating leukemia was one of the top scientists in the country and had helped develop the treatment. They spent months studying the situation and finally decided to go ahead with it. "I knew in my mind I was O.K., but I wasn't absolutely sure the cancer wouldn't come back. The considerations were: the pain I would have to undergo again, the possibility of infection and the fact that I was already much better," Doug said. But he still hadn't ruled out the treatment. After all, they got me into a remission the first time. They did save my life. So back to Mary Hitchcock he went for another harvest which is still being kept frozen in the event the cancer returns. "I just hope I never have to use it," he said.

Looking back on the past nine years of his illness, Doug sees that getting sick actually changed his life in many positive ways. "I am a stronger, better person now. I see myself as more sensitive and understanding and less directed at unimportant things. I used to have a difficult time expressing my feelings, and was a standoffish father. Now I spend more time with my children. I hug them regularly and let them know that I love them and how much they mean to me," he said. While his career and personal achievements are still a top priority, they are secondary to the time he now spends with his family and taking care of himself. Doug says he worked too much and too intensely, took himself too seriously, even at play, and didn't get enough quality time with his family. While still very active, he now tries to balance his life more with quiet time and less intensity in work and play.

What could have caused his cancer? Doug doesn't really know, but he suspects all the stress in his life plus a diet high in meat, fats, sugar and chemicals. With such a hectic work schedule, meals were often hurried or taken on the run. Breakfast was typically bacon and eggs or French toast and milk; lunch was generally a hamburger or hotdog, and dinner was either steak, lamb, roast beef or chicken with frozen or canned vegetables. Meals were served with plenty of bread and butter, and Doug's favorite beverage, milk, which he drank daily in large quantities. Dessert usually consisted of a brownie, pudding or fruit, which he usually liked to save until bedtime. Prior to his current job, he spent two years in a position which was not suited to him. He was unhappy for much of that time and unfulfilled at work and at home. "In addition, my wife and I were having marital difficulties so my life was not at it's best," Doug recalled.

In addition to the stress, Doug also wonders about the significance of his contact with a powerful chemical he used several years ago while trying to rid his home of ants. Also, ironically, a friend of his who served with him in the Army, died of leukemia five years after leaving the service.

Now that he is on a macrobiotic diet, Doug feels that the changes in his diet, along with his positive thinking and visualizations, were the key to his healing. The food was purifying his body as his mind was mentally healing it, according to him. "I had to learn to like the food, of course, which took a while for me. But what kept me on track was the realization that eating that way was better than shots in the rear and vomiting. I believe that the diet was doing the job the chemicals did at one time and couldn't do now," he said.

A typical day for Doug starts at 6:00 A.M. where you can find him in the kitchen starting miso soup and the day's grain. He then does a half hour of yoga, rides his stationary bicycle and has breakfast before going to work. He still plays hard at golf, biking, aerobics or skiing, but he finds a balance by not "working" at it and doing some calming activities like yoga and visualizations.

Nancy found the transition into macrobiotics much easier than her husband. She had an interest in the holistic way of life for many years and taught yoga and studied natural cooking. At first Doug and Nancy shared the preparation of meals, but two years ago Nancy decided to take time off from cooking and veered away from macrobiotics. After following a weight loss program for a number of months, she developed pneumonia, and subsequently went off that diet. She is now back into eating macrobiotically again, and Doug hopes she'll want to get back into cooking again since he finds her to be a better cook and more creative in the kitchen than he is.

A lot of people may start on a macrobiotic diet, Doug and Nancy have found, but leave it because it isn't easy, fast and simple. They want to do it but are easily discouraged and give up, unwilling to make the sacrifices necessary to maintain it. Sometimes it takes an illness like Doug's to force people to change their thinking and ways of eating and living, they say. "It's difficult when you don't have support. The diet can be tough and demanding at first. You need a strong will and lots of support to continue eating this way, and once you've conquered it, you've got to be careful about what you eat so you don't keep going out of balance," according to Doug. Most people think macrobiotics makes a lot of sense when I tell them about it," says Doug. "It is simple, practical and easy to understand. The practice of chewing food well, understanding the purpose of our teeth and the length of our intestines and how they all work point to the direction of a macrobiotic way of eating. Using gas cooking with a real flame to energize the food makes sense, too. It is more feasible than using electricity or microwaves for cooking.

When the Blampieds started taking cooking classes and studying macrobiotics, they decided it would be fun and helpful for them to host some classes of their own. They invited some of the teachers from the Kushi Institute to their home to lecture about the macrobiotic way of life and offered cooking classes on a weekly basis. In addition, Doug occasionally speaks to groups and organizations about his remarkable story.

Doug hasn't let his new way of life get in the way of his work. While he does find it difficult to be at a stressful eight-hour day and then come home to cook, he maintains it is worth the time and effort. He takes his lunch to work every day and when traveling, carries his food in a suitcase. He'll take things with him such as nori rolls, sourdough bread, bancha tea and natural snacks.

A year ago Doug's company had a big convention scheduled at

the Hyatt Hotel in Cambridge. Six thousand people were to attend and lunch was to be served. Without letting anyone know of his special dietary needs, Doug received a letter from the head chef at the office in New Jersey that was preparing the food for the event. The chef explained that he knew Doug was on a special diet and was willing to cook a meal just for him. To Doug's surprise, he discovered that the chef was macrobiotic too, even though he cooked conventional foods for a living. "I have found that it is all right to be aggressive about your dietary needs. When I go to restaurants I explain, 'Look, I don't want butter on my food; I want it cooked plain. I want steamed vegetables, rice and a little fish,' and I usually can get my needs met," said Doug.

Nancy said she learned that you have to put all the pieces together if you want to become macrobiotic. "You can't play at it and expect it to work. You have to do it all or don't do it. Don't dabble in it if you're trying to recover your health. Stick to it carefully until you get results, then you can broaden out a bit," she said. Doug recommended that anyone seeking to begin macrobiotics get involved in a support group and philosophy classes. He said that people have to understand why they are eating the food so they can appreciate how it is helping them. "Don't do it just because Michio says it's what you're supposed to do," he said.

The sequence of events that led Doug into a macrobiotic way of life was critical in keeping him on the path. "By meeting with John Mann, hearing Michio speak that evening, running into the man at the lecture who had healed his leukemia, going for the Way of Life Seminar weekend, and taking cooking and philosophy classes everything fell neatly into place for me." He says he is grateful for the help John Mann was able to provide during his crisis. Nancy agreed with Doug's remarks, "He was available when we had any questions or problems. There were times when we really got scared, and we needed someone to talk to. John was always there for us."

Now that he has good health, Doug finds it harder to be as careful with his diet as he'd like to be. His binge foods are chips and beer, and he "cheats by eating in the evening before he goes to bed." He has been told that this is a common habit among leukemia patients. Since he is healthy now, he doesn't feel the need to be as strict with his diet; however, should the cancer ever return, he said he'd go back to his basic macrobiotic diet again immediately.

One advantage to eating macrobioticaly is that it allows me to eat all the food I want and not gain any weight," Doug remarked. "I used to be a very big eater. To work it off, I'd have to be very vigorous. At the most I weighed 165 pounds, which, while not extremely heavy, alway felt too big for me." At his thinnest, Doug weighed in at 122 pounds. This was when he was still very weak and recovering from cancer. He and Nancy became concerned that the macrobiotic diet might not be helping, but John Mann encouraged them to stay on track and assured him that he'd gain back the weight. "He was right," Doug confirmed, "I've stabilized my weight now at about 145 pounds. Maintaining a macrobiotic way of life has been fairly easy for Doug, since he saw such immediate results from changing his "meat and potatoes" fare. "My cancer count dropped almost immediately and stayed down. That was a pretty good incentive to learn to like the food." He does think, however, that it might not be as easy for someone to make the transition if he doesn't notice immediate results. "I got a phone call the other day from a man in Ohio who has been on the diet for about five months. He is feeling discouraged because he isn't noticing any significant changes yet. I can imagine that must be a very difficult situation. Fortunately, that wasn't the case for me." Doug said he sometimes thinks to himself, "Am I going to do this for the rest of my life? The same answer keeps coming back — yes."

The program that was outlined for Doug by Michio Kushi and John Mann included not only dietary recommendations, but also many lifestyle suggestions including regular exercise, rest, chewing well, time and volume of eating, body scrubbing, cooking tips and many other concepts inherent in a healthy, balanced macrobiotic way of life.

Doug learned that in order to thoroughly maximize the healing benefits of whole natural food, proper chewing was necessary. According to Michio Kushi, whole grains and other complex carbohydrates are broken down largely in the mouth through interaction with saliva. By chewing well, the digestive process occurs smoothly and efficiently and nutrients are absorbed more effectively. It allows us to get by with less food because we utilize it more effectively. Improperly digested foods are often inefficiently absorbed so we get less nutritional benefit from what we eat, and these foods often stagnate in the body, causing a buildup of mucus and fat. These accumulations can often lead to health problems such as cysts, tumors or stones, and in some cases diseases such as cancer, arthritis and heart disease.

Doug admits that he was a gulper before learning how to chew his food well. Nancy accused him of not being able to count to 100, since after thirty or forty chews, he would find it hard to not stop there and swallow his food. Through macrobiotics, Doug learned to pay attention to his eating, which for him meant slowing down, and having an appreciation and loving feeling for what he was putting in his mouth.

Food was to be eaten preferably in a relaxed, calm manner, without a lot of conversation or distraction. This allowed the concentration on chewing and prevented Doug from bolting his food or swallowing food whole. The use of chopsticks was encouraged for Doug since they prevented him from putting too much food in his mouth at one time, and wood is more natural for eating than metal.

Doug was advised to have meals regularly, two to three times per day, and to avoid eating for approximately three hours before sleeping. Michio says that if we eat too soon before going to sleep, our food will not digest properly and can stagnate in the intestines. This can lead to inefficient absorption and often unnecessary weight gain. If we don't eat before sleeping, he said we have much more peaceful and restful sleep, and our bodies are able to wake up thoroughly refeshed and renewed. It is much easier to get up the following morning refreshed to pursue the day's challenges with full vigor. Going to bed with a full stomach often disturbs our sleep so that we may feel tired and sluggish the next morning. For optimum health, Michio recommends only bancha tea and other moderate beverages if one feels the need to have something in the stomach before bedtime.

Doug confesses that he still has a hard time avoiding eating at night. He used to eat brownies or cookies and now eats macrobiotic cookies, pie or other desserts. He says he tries very hard not to eat too late and is successful at times, but isn't always. He also says he tries not to be too hard on himself when he isn't doing the right thing.

Doug was advised to scrub his body daily with a hot towel to activate and improve the circulation of his blood and body fluids. According to Michio, many illnesses are furthered by poor circulation, which deprives cells of nutrients carried by the blood and can allow a buildup of toxins. Body scrubbing, as well as other forms of moderate exercise, helps release these stagnations and accumulations. This is especially true in the case of leukemia and other illnesses of the blood, says Michio.

A second benefit of body scrubbing is to open and expand the pores of the skin so that excess fats, minerals and other waste products can be discharged more efficiently. After many years of consuming meat, chicken, cheese, eggs and dairy products which contain hard saturated fat, a layer of hard fat often builds up just beneath the skin. In this blocked condition, toxins can easily build up in the bloodstream and internal organs and contribute to the development of serious illness. Michio suggested that Doug avoid taking hot baths or showers, as these can deplete valuable minerals from the body and cause us to become tired or fatigued. He suggested we take quick, moderately hot showers or baths when necessary.

All that is needed for a body scrub, Doug was told, is a sink with hot water and a medium-sized cotton towel. Hold the towel at either end and place it under a stream of hot water. Wring out the towel, and while it is still hot and steamy, begin to scrub with it, beginning with hands and fingers, and working the way up the arms to the shoulders, neck and face, and then downward to the chest, upper back, abdomen, lower back, buttocks, legs, feet and toes. The scrubbing should continue until the skin turns slightly red or until each part becomes warm, about ten minutes total for the whole body. As the towel starts to cool, reheat it again by running it under hot water after finishing each section of the body.

Doug found the body scrubbing to be relaxing and invigorating and liked the way it helped relieve the stress and tension particularly after a hard day at work. He was advised especially to do a ginger body scrub, with the addition of fresh ginger root to the pot of hot water. Doug found this method more convenient on weekends when he had more time. He was instructed to take a golfball-size piece of grated ginger and put it into a cheesecloth sack to be dipped in the hot water. Without boiling, he simmered the ginger for a few minutes then used that for the scrubbing water. One pot of hot ginger water could be used for two days of body scrubs. The water could be simply reheated and used again.

Michio suggested a regular program of light to moderate exercise to restore vitality and energy levels. He advised Doug to choose a form of exercise that suited his needs and make it a part of his daily routine. He especially recommended walking as a convenient form of non-strenuous exercise. A half-hour walk each day was recommended, regardless of the weather. Doug bought a stationary bicycle and did a fifteen-minute workout every day as well as a walk around the block at his home. He found it to be boring, but knew that it was part of the healing process. One thing he noticed was that he didn't have to go for pain in being the fastest or the best. His bicycling and walking was not competitive as most of his prior activities had been. He said that prior to getting sick he always felt the need to do more. For the first year of his healing program, he discontinued his regular sports and only walked, biked or performed yoga exercises.

When it came to cooking, Doug and Nancy had no trouble converting from electric to gas cooking, especially after hearing Michio's recommendations. Michio says that electricity dissipates the molecular structure and strength of food by causing the electrons to bounce out of the atomic field, leaving the atom very unstable. Gas, on the other hand, just bounces the molecules around, while leaving them intact. In addition, electricity makes it difficult to cook uniformly and it is possible that the ingredients at the bottom of the pan can burn while those at the top need more cooking. A gas flame has the surrounding air, and thus food cooks much more evenly. Also, the temperature can be adjusted immediately, and meals are more well cooked. A microwave oven should be avoided, particularly if a family member is sick. These ovens zap food with radioactive waves at three-billion-cycles per second (an electric stove runs at 60-cycles per second and actually generates a low form of radiation). It disintegrates food instead of cooking it and can cause the same effect in our body. Microwave cooking cannot help in regaining health, and it is suspected to contribute to certain types of illness, according to Michio. Because of these drawbacks in electric and microwave cooking, a person may not feel satisfied with the meal and may crave strong salt or animal food to counter the weakening effects, which in turn causes a craving for excessive sweets. Michio found that those who shifted to gas cooking from electricity had reported such benefits as improved energy levels, increased appetite and enjoyment of food.

In addition to learning about basic dietary recommendations, Doug needed help with a "sweet tooth," which he learned was caused by overeating foods such as chicken, cheese, eggs, shellfish and others that cause hard fats to accumulate in the pancreas. This fat interferes with the secretion of glycogen or anti-insulin, a hormone that normally raises the level of glucose, or sugar in the blood to within the normal range. Insulin, which is complementary to glycogen, lowers the blood sugar level.

The symptoms of tiredness, chronic fatigue, depression and craving for sweets are often a sign of hypoglycemia, or low blood sugar, according to Michio. The symptoms occur most frequently in the late afternoon or early evening, when the blood sugar dips below normal. To overcome these symptoms, most people will reach for chocolate, a soft drink or a cup of coffee with sugar in it. The problem with this form of energy is that the simple sugars in these foods are rapidly absorbed into the bloodstream and burned up quickly, resulting in the blood sugar going below normal in a short period of time, and creating the original symptoms of fatigue and depletion of energy.

Doug was advised to provide his body with plenty of complex carbohydrates, especially in the form of whole grains, beans and sweet tasting vegetables, which would provide an excellent source of energy without producing extremes in the blood sugar levels. It was suggested that Doug take a sweet vegetable drink for a month or so until his symptoms of hypoglycemia began to diminish. To prepare this drink, he was told to cut equal amounts of carrots, onions, butternut squash and green cabbage into very fine pieces and boil with four times the amount of water for ten to fifteen minutes. The liquid was then strained through a fine mesh strainer into a large glass jar, which could be stored in the refrigerator for several days. Doug was told that the drink could be used daily to relieve the craving for sugar and other sweets and to restore energy and vitality.

Michio advised against wearing any synthetic fibers such as polyester, nylon or rayon against the skin. He said that sythetics interfere with the exchange of energy between the body and surrounding environment and contribute to a feeling of tiredness and fatigue. He recommended that Doug wear cotton and other natural vegetable quality fabrics, especially in undergarments and any other garment that came in direct contact with the skin. He further recommended the use of cotton towels, sheets and pillowcases.

Doug was told to limit the time he spent watching television or operating a computer since these devices emit various forms of radiation and could weaken his condition and slow his recovery. He was advised to place green plants throughout his house to refresh and enrich the oxygen content of the air. And, somewhat humorously, Michio suggested he sing a happy song every day in order to help him breathe more deeply and elevate his mood and spirits.

Finally, Michio mentioned that an important aspect of healing was to relax mentally and physically and to live each day happily without being preoccupied by health concerns. He suggested Doug develop an "attitude of gratitude" for nature, his friends, family and all people he encountered, and his daily food, including enjoying it thoroughly. An important aspect of this was to have enough variety in his cooking and daily meals. "Food should be interesting and delicious," Michio said. "If it is dull or tasteless, we can't enjoy it and will not be healthy or happy."

Part II
Personal Accounts

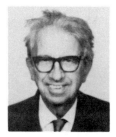

6

Hugh Faulkner, M.D.
Pancreatic Cancer

My surgeon has asked me to talk today about my own experience of macrobiotics, and some of my ideas on how to bring two worlds closer together: complementary medicine and orthodox Western medicine.

First my own experience. I retired in 1976 and moved to Italy, after nearly thirty years as a general practitioner in North London. More by luck than by good management, I had bought a peasant farmhouse in the middle of Chianti just before the property boom. Then, I managed to get taken on as a part-time consultant in primary health care to the Tuscan region and the local health district in the new Italian health service. Some of our friends think that voluntarily getting involved with the setting up of two national health services in a span of thirty years is the height of masochism. My wife, Marian, who had been a nurse in general practice for a smaller number of years, was brave enough to come along as well, and we have been living very happily in Italy for nearly fourteen years.

Just after Christmas in early 1987, I consulted Dr. Beck at a London hospital, on the advice of my old friend, Professor Exton Smith. I had had persistent diarrhea for several years and more recently a loss of weight. A thorough investigation some eight years before at another hospital had revealed no abnormality, and I had almost accepted the label "irritable colon." Almost, but not quite, because I was happier than I had ever been, with no obvious evidence of stress. Routine investigations at the Whittington Hospital in London also were normal, until an observant radiologist spotted a possible filling defect in my barium enema. A subsequent ultrasound revealed a mass in the region of the head of the pancreas. The next day my surgeon, John Cochrane, advised an operation as soon as possible. When Marian, assuming that I had a cancer which was likely to be inoperable, asked what would happen if I didn't have the operation, Mr. Cochrane said that I would almost certainly obstruct. Naturally I decided to have the operation.

I gather that pancreatic cancer is now one of the leading causes of death from cancer and appears to be on the increase, so many of you have probably seen more cases than I have. The most up-to-date information I have seen is in a very thorough report by Gudjonsson who reviewed 196 cases of proved carcinoma of the pancreas seen at Yale New Haven Hospital during the ten years from 1972 to 1982. The mean survival from the date of diagnosis for the patient group as a whole was 208 days, about seven months. Twenty-seven patients lived for more than one year, ten for two years, four for three years and only one for more than five years. He died in the sixth year. No spontaneous regressions were reported in the hospital series. As you know, unsubstantiated claims have been made for the use of chemotherapy and radiotherapy. Resection, the Whipple's operation of my youth, is seldom performed today in Britain, though I am told that it is still attempted in some parts of the United States. Tamoxifen, which has had some success in breast cancer and conflicting reports for pancreatic cancer, is the subject of a large controlled clinical trial in Norway which I haven't seen reported yet. In fact, there appears to be no convincing evidence that any orthodox treatment affects the prognosis. Gudjonsson concludes that "40 percent of those found to have cancer of the pancreas will be dead within three months, 65 percent within six months, and close to 90 percent within one year from the time of diagnosis." You will not be surprised to learn that I booked a bed in a hospice, of which we have had good reports. We had begun to wonder whether an isolated Tuscan peasant farmhouse was the most convenient place to die in.

John Cochrane operated some four or five days after the ultrasound. He told me that he found a tumor the size of a cricket ball in the head of the pancreas, with no evidence of spread. No attempt was made to resect the tumor but a double bypass was done. A biopsy subsequently confirmed an adenocarcinoma (tumor of a gland).

I was very impressed to find physicians and surgeons actively cooperating in the gastrointestinal unit and I was very well looked after. However, I was disappointed that I had no advice on postoperative rehabilitation or diet. Perhaps an ex-GP [General Practioner] was supposed to know it all. I think we all tend to forget that patients with an inoperable cancer and their relatives could be helped to improve the quality of their remaining weeks or months, by social workers, dietitians and physiotherapists. We, of course, were privileged with a great deal of support from family and friends, but I still wanted to recover as far as possible from the laparotomy (surgical procedure in which an incision is made into the abdominal wall), and thought some rehabilitation might help.

Marian and I had experimented with shiatsu massage from a book we had bought, and found it helpful in treating muscle pain. Shiatsu, for those not familiar with it, is a very old Oriental system of massage based on similar principles to acupuncture, but using the hands, and sometimes feet, knees, and elbows, instead of needles. At the Community Health Foundation, in Old Street, I contacted Hilary Totah, a leading shiatsu expert. She came to the house where I was staying after my discharge from the hospital and gave me shiatsu massage which immediately relieved a lot of the pain and stiffness. Just as she was going she said, "You do know that shiatsu doesn't relieve cancer, don't you? But have you thought about macrobiotics? I could arrange for you to see someone at the Community Health Foundation if you like." I said that I had never heard of macrobiotics and would rather read about it before meeting an enthusiastic believer. On her next visit she brought me a book on macrobiotics and Marian bought another in Compendium bookshop, in Camden Town.

Here, for the first time, was someone offering hope — if not of cure, at least the possibility of doing something which might help. For us, macrobiotics was a completely new idea. We discussed it with friends and relatives and with my physician. We decided I had nothing to lose and just possibly everything to gain. But on the advice of another old friend, before actually embarking on macrobiotics we consulted with a GP who founded the British Holistic Medical Association. He confirmed that macrobiotics was a perfectly respectable and responsible discipline but warned us that he knew of no evidence, other than anecdotal, that macrobiotics could relieve an established cancer of the pancreas. When Marian asked him if he would try macrobiotics if he was in my position, he said, "Probably not!"

Despite this rather lukewarm recommendation, we decided to go ahead and booked a private interview with Jon Sandifer, a leading macrobiotic teacher, whose father was a GP who qualified in the same year I did. Jon was held up elsewhere and arranged for us to see Edward Esko, a delightful, extroverted American from Boston who was a visiting lecturer, and is very well known in the macrobiotic world. Edward was convinced that I could recover and gave us preliminary advice on diet and way of life, but strongly advised us to have cooking lessons, to continue with shiatsu massage, and to see Michio Kushi, the founder of the Kushi Institute in Boston, while he was still in Europe. So we took his advice.

We arranged to see Michio Kushi in France on our way back to Italy. He was addressing a conference of French doctors at Bergerac, which provided a very good introduction to macrobiotics. Michio is Japanese and speaks with a strong accent. He is quiet and modest and discourages attempts to make him a guru or a saint. During the meeting I asked him if macrobiotics could relieve my cancer. "No" he replied, "but your body can!" He recommended a standard macrobiotic diet with adjustments for my condition, mainly based on 50-60 percent brown rice and other whole grains, cooked green vegetables, root vegetables, such as turnips and and carrots, and seaweed from Japan. Meat, fish, alcohol, refined sugar, baked flour products including bread, cakes, and biscuits, were to be avoided. One of our friends calls this the "No No" diet because whenever you ask whether you can eat anything the answer is always "No!"

I had two further meetings with Michio. At the second one, four months later, he told me I was much better, which was immensely reassuring, because I did in fact feel very well. On this occasion Michio suggested I write a book about my story with the help of Marian and my shiatsu teacher in Florence who had studied with Michio in Boston. We have just completed the first draft of the book, entitled *Beating The Odds*, and our agent in Rome is looking for Italian and American publishers.

After our return to Italy, I continued to make a rapid recovery. I still take the pancreatic enzyme, the hormone Tamoxifen, folic acid and cimetidine prescribed by my hospital consultants. Four months after the operation I was swimming twenty lengths in the local baths. This improvement has been maintained. My weight remains constant at 65 kilos, and I have more energy than I have had for years. I am involved in writing two books. I am busy trying to raise money in our health district in Chianti for a research project on prevention.

In all this activity Marian has played a vital role. She had been vegetarian for several years and is a theosophist, and found it easier to accept the underlying philosophy, diet, and lifestyle than I did. In fact she is much more meticulous about the diet than I am and regards Michio's words as divine law. But without Marian's help, love and understanding it would all have been very, very much more difficult.

I would now like to forget about the cancer and concentrate on seeing how fit I can be at the age of seventy-five. George Ohsawa, the founder of modern macrobiotics, used to say: "Congratulations. You've got cancer! Now you can start a new life!" I hope I have.

Today, well over two years after the initial diagnosis, I feel extremely well. I can't claim conclusively that my cancer is regressing, though ultrasound and a CT scan suggest some shrinking and liquefaction in the center of the tumor area. Nor can I prove that my present state is the result of macrobiotics. This story is just another example of the anecdotal accounts many physicians quite properly find unconvincing. However it has persuaded me that further dialogue is desirable between orthodox Western medical science and complementary medicine. The situation in the States where both sides appear to hurl insults at one another across a Berlin Wall of misunderstanding is deplorable.

In Britain, increasing numbers of people appear to be turning to complementary medicine. The editor of the *Journal of Alternative and Complementary Medicine* tells me that they list over fifty national bodies in this field, but that is almost certainly an underestimate. They hear of new organizations every few days, mostly offshoots of American ventures. Some twelve centers are listed as carrying out research. Eight organizations are concerned with holistic medicine. There is an all-party parliamentary committee on complementary medicine. Recent articles in the medical press suggest that the majority of GPs in Britain are now prepared to refer patients to practitioners in complementary medicine when they think that it could help. A small survey carried out by National Opinion Polls for the City Health Centre of people living and working in the City reported recently in the *Guardian* found that most respondents viewed complementary medicine as effective. Two out of three people would like to see it available on the national health service and four out of five would like it on private health insurance. It is obvious that the scene has changed completely since we left Britain some thirteen years ago.

The diet in macrobiotics is regarded as very important, but it is only one side of the total picture. We have found in macrobiotics, in London, in Florence, and at the summer camp at Lenk in Switzerland last year, a warm supportive atmosphere of hope and positive thinking which has been of great help to us both. We have met many people with widely differing backgrounds and beliefs. Many of them are firmly convinced that macrobiotics has helped them to overcome a major illness or a chronic condition.

So what are the obstacles to the further recognition and acceptance of macrobiotics? First, if macrobiotics wants to be taken seriously by orthodox medicine it has got to take itself seriously. It is no answer to say that many of the things we do as doctors have never been submitted to double-blind controlled clinical trials. Macrobiotic teachers will have to keep accurate records even if most GPs don't. There should be a standardized questionnaire and record card for all the Kushi Institutes. On my suggestion Michio Kushi has sent material to an epidemiologist in the World Health Organization with a request for advice on possible epidemiological studies, in which some of us would be prepared to take part. Although some research workers are narrowly orthodox, others are not, and I believe that serious studies would be taken seriously by a good research unit or most medical journals.

Next, if it does work, how does it work? Macrobiotics is based on traditional Far Eastern medicine, and was developed in its modern form by the Japanese philosopher, George Ohsawa. He used its methods to cure himself of tuberculosis in the early part of this century before we had effective chemotherapy. It has been carried on by his students, of whom Michio Kushi is the best known. It is still based on the principles of yin and yang, as George Ohsawa puts it in his book, on a dialectical approach. I was exposed to dialectics as a student and have no difficulties in the concept of yin and yang as complementary opposites, changing into one another in a world of continuous motion. Nor do these ideas seem far removed from recent advances in physics, as I understand them from popular books and articles, though very different from the mechanistic Cartesian science I was taught fifty years ago.

Nor is it difficult to accept the classification of foods and organs of the body as predominantly yin or yang. Ohsawa said that there is yin acid forming food, yang acid forming food, yin alkaline forming food and yang alkaline forming food, referring to the pH of the blood. But as far as I know no one has demonstrated how the diet could have a direct effect on individual cells, which could explain why macrobiotics believe that certain foods cause cancer and that others relieve it.

A young German, Reinhold Solch, has kindly sent me a copy of a paper he read at the annual conference of macrobiotic teachers at Kiental in Switzerland. I am not competent to understand all its implications or to make any assessment of its validity, but he appears to have made a heroic search of the literature on intracellular pH. Solch quotes recent work suggesting that intracellular pH plays an important role in tumor growth, which he believes could explain how foods could cause, prevent, or relieve cancer. If Solch's hypothesis is correct, it could provide a scientific explanation for what appears to have happened to me and everyone else on a macrobiotic diet. Solch is a computer expert and not a biologist. We are arranging for someone in cancer research to have a look at his paper.

Further, how do acupuncture and shiatsu work? Most people who have had these treatments are convinced that they do something, but what? I have only had acupuncture on one occasion, with some benefit to an acute back condition, the day before I was running a conference! But I have had shiatsu on many occasions, and have experienced very different reactions to different operators and different techniques. Both acupuncture and shiatsu are based on the concept of Ki and the meridians, but as far as I know no one has yet demonstrated either by accepted scientific methods. Ki in Japanese means "the life force." In China it is called *Ch'i*, and in India, *Prana*. It is found in all the Eastern traditional medicines, and the concept must be several thousand years old. Ki is believed to travel along the meridians which are illustrated on the colorful charts often displayed by practitioners of both acupuncture and shiatsu.

However, in their recent book *The Dark Side of the Brain*, Oldfield and Coghill report some revolutionary theories which they claim have a scientific basis. They postulate that each organic cell has a unique radio frequency determined and controlled by the cerebral cortex. Each cell's resonant frequency helps to control the organic form of the whole organism. As a result of Kirlian photography and electromagnetic research, mainly in Rumania, but also in the USA and Britain, experimental support is said to be emerging for this hypothesis. Once again I am not competent to make any kind of critical assessment of these claims, and can only report what is inevitably causing great interest in the rather restricted macrobiotic circles we move in. It seems clear that a great deal more research is required before this thesis can be proved or disproved. However, this work could have obvious relevance for acupuncture, shiatsu, the meridians and the existence of Ki. Indeed Carpenter believes that he has recorded Ki with Kirlian photography, and demonstrated an aura round the heads of certain people, and not only the saints in medieval paintings. I must confess that I would welcome explanations of my personal experience of macrobiotics along acceptable scientific lines, without postulating entirely new phenomena or old and mysterious forces from the East.

Few of us would disagree with the macrobiotic emphasis on physical exercise, relaxation, fresh air, and pure water. I believe that all systems of complementary medicine have these in common. I have no personal experience of yoga or meditation, and they were not directly recommended in my case. Many macrobiotics practice one or both, although they are clearly not confined to macrobiotics. There is a vast literature on them; they are said to be increasingly practiced in Britain, and I imagine that there is plenty of evidence that they help some people. Perhaps the medical profession should know more about them.

One of the most important gifts macrobiotics gave me in the early days was the feeling that I had regained control of my own body, perhaps of my own destiny. Macrobiotics believe that all illness is due to an imbalance in our rapport with nature, and that in most cases we have it in our power to correct this by the food we eat and our way of life. Human beings, once supplied with the basic necessities of life, have almost infinite capacity for growth and change. This view is shared by many of the various human potential movements, quasi-religious sects and self-help groups.

A major problem is that macrobiotics is outside the health service, and therefore reserved for those who can afford to pay privately for cooking classes and other educational services, chromium steel pans, various Japanese products and natural whole foods. At the international camp at Lenk in Switzerland last year we saw no one obviously poor. Yet if macrobiotics can be shown to be effective in preventing and relieving cancer and some other diseases it should be available to all.

Lastly, a problem I have met among those practicing macrobiotics, and indeed others who follow Eastern philosophical beliefs is the deep opposition to collective action — the conviction, shared by the medical establishment, that we should keep out of politics. Many of our macrobiotic friends are prepared to talk about violence, about pollution, the chemicalization of our foods, the use of herbicides and pesticides, deforestation, and all the other crimes against nature committed for immediate financial gain. They often sign their letters "Yours, in love and peace," yet they studiously avoid taking part in any action which could help people to resist these things. I firmly believe that the ecology movement and the organizations like Physicians Against War can have a major influence on politicians and events. Everyone involved in orthodox medicine or complementary medicine should play a part in these movements, however small. If we genuinely want peace, natural food uncontaminated by chemicals, clean air and water, we should be prepared to do something about it.

Orthodox Western medicine has a great deal to learn from complementary medicine — and from macrobiotics in particular. They could learn about health promotion, prevention, diet, exercise, lifestyle, about developing the fullest potential of our minds and bodies, about self-help — particularly when orthodox medicine has nothing more to offer.

I believe that many people in complementary medicine need to know more about what is good in orthodox medicine and not only what is bad. They need to know about some of the genuine advances, about recent work in psychotherapy, about evaluation, self-audit and peer audit, and some of the important developments in our own field. I am not urging you to send all your patients to macrobiotic teachers. I don't know if my experience is repeatable. I have simply tried to take you along some of the roads I have traveled during the past two years and am asking you to keep an open mind.

I've learned quite a bit about macrobiotics in the past two years, and quite a bit about myself. In my years of general practice I have learned that nothing, absolutely nothing, can be ruled out in medicine. I am convinced that complementary medicine is helping some people with problems we have not solved. What would I do about it if I was still in general practice in Camden? I would certainly be happy to cooperate with macrobiotic practitioners as I do in Italy. I believe that GPs are already working in a group practice with complementary practitioners in Marylebone. This seems an interesting development which should be encouraged, and perhaps tried in some of the health centers and other group practices. Finally, in the case of patients I couldn't help further who wanted to try macrobiotics, I hope I would give them the support and encouragement I have had from my own GP and my hospital consultants.

Source: Hugh Faulkner, M.D., "A GP Looks at Macrobiotics," based on a talk given at Whittington Hospital, London to GPs in a refresher course, June 1, 1989.

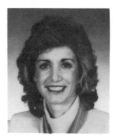

7.

Marlene McKenna
Malignant Melanoma

In 1983, Marlene McKenna was diagnosed with malignant melanoma. "As a working mother of four children, radio/TV commentator, and investment broker, I was living a very unbalanced life," Marlene explained in a recent interview in *The Providence Visitor*.

In August 1985, she began to complain of severe stomach pains, and in January 1986, doctors discovered that five tumors had spread throughout her body. Two feet of her intestines were removed, and Marlene was told she had six months to a year to live.

Declining all treatments, Marlene turned to macrobiotics at the suggestion of her brother and visited Michio Kushi in Boston. In addition to changing her diet, she brought in a gas stove in place of her electric stove, and began to meditate and practice yoga. A devout Catholic, she also did a lot of inspirational reading and praying.

"I promised God that if He walked me through this and helped me live, I would give Him life with life," she recalls.

Within a year, she was on the way to recovery, and doctors found no evidence of further cancer. Feeling well enough to return to public life, she ran for state treasurer in Rhode Island. During the campaign, she discovered that she was pregnant. Because of her previous illness and age (forty-two), doctors encouraged her to get an abortion. Marlene refused. "I realized that (having the baby) was part of my promise to give life with life," she explains. Though she lost the election, she gave birth to a healthy baby boy, keeping her promise to God and proving her physicians wrong.

Since then, she has opened a macrobiotic natural foods restaurant in Providence, Shepherd's, and is helping people around the country who have heard of her remarkable recovery.

Source: *One Peaceful World* Newsletter, Becket, Massachusetts, Autumn, 1989.

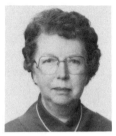

8.

Betty Metzger
Malignant Melanoma

During the month of August 1980, I underwent surgery for malignant melanoma. That consisted of removing an area about 4 1/2-inches in diameter of tissue down to the muscle on my right shoulder. Skin was grafted from my thigh. The surgery healed nicely and after a few months I felt reasonably safe that my cancer problem was solved.

However, in November 1981, there appeared a lump on the right side of my neck. The cancer had spread to the lymph nodes. My surgeon removed the cancerous nodes and during the week before Christmas 1981 I received chemotherapy for five consecutive days. There would be a three-week rest before the next regimen of five daily treatments. My oncologist said this would continue for a year at which time they would reevaluate my condition.

Chemotherapy was halted from the first of June to the end of August because of low white blood cell counts. I received the August treatments and three days of the September regimen when I felt that I could no longer go on.

A friend told me about Dr. Sattilaro's account of his survival from cancer in the August [1982] issue of *Life*. My husband and I read *Recalled By Life* by Dr. Sattilaro and Jean and Mary Alice Kohler's book *Healing Miracles From Macrobiotics*. That and my family's encouragement were all I needed to embark on a macrobiotic way of life. I sought and found much help from friends who were on the diet and read everything about it that was available.

It has now been nine years since my first cancer surgery. I feel great, thanking God every day for the precious gift of good health.

Source: Correspondence with Betty Metzger, Shelby, Ohio, August, 1989.

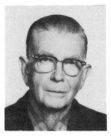

9.

Cecil Dudley
Colon Cancer

Back in 1982, when I was seventy-five, I went to an internist for a complete physical check-up. This included a sigmoidoscope of the colon but for some reason did not include the Hemoccult II slide test, which checks the feces for blood. In March 1982, several months after my last examination, I consulted my internist again regarding pain in the abdomen and he prescribed a tranquilizer for "gas."

My guardian angel must have been looking out for me when I saw a newspaper write-up about a course titled "Avoid Dying of Cancer — Now or Later" conducted once a year at Ohio State University. While it was attended primarily by approximately 300 medical and nurse students, senior citizens could attend without charge. Included in the course was the voluntary testing of the feces for blood by the Hemoccult II slide method. In the course I learned that everyone over fifty years of age should have such a check once a year. The test can be done by the individual in the privacy of his home.

My test was positive whereupon I had a barium enema which

showed a tumor in the colon. It was removed without a colostomy. One year later the results of a liver CT scan prompted me to investigate the macrobiotic diet. I learned of it from a TV newscast. It told how Dr. Anthony Sattilaro picked up two hitchhikers and learned of the diet.

I attended the Macrobiotic Way of Life Seminar in Boston to learn about cooking, home care, and macrobiotic principles. Since then I have attended four of the macrobiotic summer conferences presented in the Berkshires which are very beneficial. For a year after going on the diet, I was given a medical check-up every three months. Since then I only have to go in once a year. With the support of my wife, Margaret, many changes were made in lifestyle, the food we purchased, the way it is prepared, how we ate, and in other aspects. I increased my amount of exercise. As a result, I experienced weight control from a lowered fat intake, my cholesterol went from 219 to 137, and I feel physically and mentally more alert and good enough to take several trips a year. My CEA levels are well within the normal range, and there is no sign of a recurrence of the cancer.

Source: Correspondence with Cecil O. Dudley, Columbus, Ohio, August, 1990.

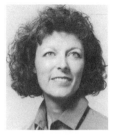

10.

Mona Sanders
Brain Cancer

In August 1986, everything was wonderful. I had just turned thirty-seven and was thoroughly enjoying life. I loved everything about it and was having a wonderful time. And then the bottom fell out.

After a grand mal seizure that sent me sprawling onto an asphalt tennis court, many, many tests in two hospitals, and two surgeries, I was diagnosed as having a grade 3 anaplastic astrocytoma. This is a fast growing inoperative brain tumor. At that time it was about the size of a small grapefruit.

Tumor . . . Tumor . . . — the name kept jumping out at me like a 3-D movie — visible, but unable to grasp. Through all of the discussions of the abnormality, tumor or cancer had never been a possibility in my mind. The reality hit home when I was asked to visit a tumor center for discussion of possible treatments for "my" brain tumor — "my" cancer.

To say that the discovery that I had cancer was an earthshaking experience was an understatement. I think the impact of the diagnosis caused me, one night soon after, to experience a series of physical jolts: nausea, vomiting, and numbness in my right leg. The emotional trauma was something that I was not accustomed to.

I've always been a contented happy person, able to see the bright side of things, even while "bitching." I could find contentment sitting on a rock at Smith Lake or in my husband's arms dancing in romantic places like Bermuda. I had always enjoyed life, living by my own decisions — until now.

The doctors said it was bad — would never go away — chemotherapy could hopefully only slow its growth — was close to the motor area — I would lose motor control — wheelchair in the future — six to eighteen months to live — downhill all the way. It was worse than a Freddie Kruger nightmare. I couldn't wake up.

IT did not belong there. I wanted IT gone.

When my aunt from New Orleans suggested macrobiotics, I had no idea what she was talking about and the idea that food could make a malignancy go away was absurd. But when you have no alternative and a strong desire to live, you will do what it takes.

So, I read *Recalled By Life* by Anthony Sattilaro, as she suggested, and later read *Recovery* by Elaine Nussbaum. Elaine was a housewife, like me, but in much worse shape. I reasoned that if she could do that I could too. It did not matter that I lived in a small town in northeast Mississippi and knew no one who had even heard of macrobiotics at that time.

Before jumping right in, though, I decided I would give the American Cancer Society hotline a final check to see if there was anything else I could do. At this point I had 6,000 RADs and two treatments of chemo (PCNU). At least five more treatments were scheduled.

The volunteer's answer was, "Nothing. Good luck." The line went dead.

Through clinched teeth my reply was, "We'll see about that!"

Three days later, January 17, 1987, I was on my way to the Macrobiotic Learning Center in Brookline, Massachusetts. This beginner course was given in a home that to me, coming from Mississippi, seemed damp and chilly. I had trouble understanding the various foreign teachers and the fast-talking Yankee instructors, and, of course, they couldn't understand my Southern accent. The ingredients for the meals could have come from another planet, and I had trouble eating and enjoying the food.

At that time, I was on many anti-seizure pills and my thinking was clouded to say the least. Luckily, I took my camcorder and taped everything, because trying to absorb everything sent me to bed with a headache each night.

In short, this was not a pleasant experience, but to come back to Columbus, and say this, I would not do. This was my chance to live and I was going to take it.

Looking back now I am able to realize how much I absorbed and credit much of my success to that program. I learned not only the proper way to cook, but also exercises, massage, home remedies, and the power of positive thinking.

So back to Columbus, Mississippi, I came, ready to get under way with my new macrobiotic life. After unpacking all the videos I'd made and the books and tapes I'd purchased, I was ready to begin. I was quick to learn that cooking alone was quite different than with an ever-ready teacher plus six other students in the kitchen. I started my first solo macro meal at 3:00 P.M. I finished a little after 8:00 P.M., at which time I was too exhausted to eat!

Another turning point came when I returned to Boston in February to see Michio Kushi. It was then that I decided to take charge of my recovery.

Taking charge meant that I was going to stop taking chemotherapy and that I was going to get off the nine anti-seizure pills and tachycardia medicine I was supposed to take for the rest of my life.

I had to tell the neuro-oncologist and my husband, David, about my decision to discontinue the chemo, but the anti-seizure medication had to be gradually decreased, and I didn't want to tell them until I had been off it and the tachycardia pills for a month. This took a year and when I told them what I had done, they had a fit. But all's been well.

Well — almost all: That first winter, my mind was so drugged that I couldn't get from the cookbook to the stove without forgetting what to do. I kept feeling worse and worse and colder and colder. But I said six months I'd try it and six months it was going to be.

From somewhere came the idea of a macrobiotic cook. After

numerous calls to our friend in Boston, John Carter, and reference checks, Dawn Gilmour arrived from Boston, and some of the food actually started tasting good!

Dawn gave me some concoctions I'd read about but never tried. One, a simple drink made with heated apple juice and diluted kuzu, had a wonderful calming effect. Dawn was a normal person with hopes, dreams, and fears like the rest of us, which meant I could identify with her, yet at the same time could learn from her.

The only regret I have was that during the week Dawn was there I would get terribly tired during meal preparation and would end up taking a nap. I don't know if this was a defense mechanism or what, but thank the Lord for Mamie.

Mamie was a wonderful woman who I'm sure was sent to me from God. In fact before she came to work for us, I was in a dither getting ready for Dawn's arrival and as always was running out of time and energy. As I stood in our breakfast room I said, "Lord, what am I going to do?"

Mamie rang the doorbell to introduce herself to me. (I had hired her a few days earlier sight unseen.) She had been on the way to town and had just decided to stop. I promptly hugged her and started crying. She then came into the house in her town clothes and helped me prepare for Dawn.

Of course, Mamie was there for Dawn's teaching and absorbed it all. Mamie had a superb memory and was a wonderful cook.

She also was like a mother to me because she would make me sit down and plan the day's menu, making sure I was eating all I was supposed to and getting the rest I needed. I truly do not know what I would have done without her guidance and persistence.

Macrobiotics was a challenge for me. Slowly, through training by the experts and experimenting on my own, I learned that I could make delicious meals that would enable me to enjoy the food while my body was healing itself.

I stopped the chemotherapy after the third treatment and began a full time holistic regime to heal my body and soul.

A verse from Ephesians in the Bible became my motto: "Now unto Him that is able to do exceedingly abundantly above all that we ask or think, according to the power that worketh in us."

God had given me the power to take charge of my life again and to make myself well. Besides prayer and macrobiotics, I used imaging. I also used a video tape and a subliminal cassette that constantly told me the tumor was decreasing. In my bedroom, I kept a drawing of the tumor that showed it decreasing in size — from the size of a grapefruit to a golfball to a pinhead to nothing! Amazingly, each test showed the malignancy diminished just as I had drawn.

The CT scan made in April of 1987, four months after starting macrobiotics, showed no evidence of cancer! And none have since then, either.

One night two years ago, my nine-year-old son, Parker, asked, "Mom, do you think you'll ever get cancer again? My immediate reply was, "No." After a bit I came back into his bedroom and added, "But, Parker, don't worry, honey, because if I do I know what to do." He smiled and said, "We'll fight like before."

It's wonderful to have that assurance. In a way the feeling can be compared to seeing a rainbow after a storm and remembering God's promise. My healing process was not just luck. It was my strong faith in God, the many prayers sent for me and by me, my determination, a positive outlook, imaging, video and subliminal tapes, and the accurate practice of the diet.

It was also the love and support from my husband, children, family, and friends who became so close they felt like sisters. It was realizing that I, not anyone else, was responsible for my health. No one thing can control cancer, not just diet, not just radiation, not just chemotherapy. The body heals itself with God's help. I used everything else as tools.

Through all these things, I have regained my physical, mental, and spiritual health. I am alive with the chance to work, play, and love, and I want to share my experiences with others to spare them the anguish I went through and to offer an alternative to degenerative disease.

Source: Correspondence with Mona Sanders, Columbus, Mississippi, August, 1990. Copyright ©1990 Mona Sanders.

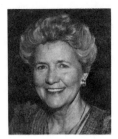

11.

Barbara Lee
Urethral Cancer

My life embarked on a new path on July 1, 1987, when the urologist, during a very painful examination, declared that he would have to take a biopsy at the hospital because my urethra contained a tumor which he was sure was malignant. He advised me to go home and talk with my family, but to enter Baylor Hospital the following Monday at 6:00 A.M.

My first reaction was disbelief, since I seemed so healthy except for this nagging pressure on my bladder, coupled with the fact that no one in my entire family had ever had cancer. I thought the doctor was probably mistaken. My husband and I were both in shock and disbelief! However, soon, I felt a deep spiritual calm and assurance that God was in control and that He would direct our path.

During the next few days, we talked and prayed with my five grown children and then with my husband's three, plus our sisters and brothers and their families. Comfort and support from close friends and family helps so much when you are devastated.

On July 3, my husband and I had lunch at our favorite health food store as we had so many times before. This time, from an open book rack, the book, *The Cancer-Prevention Diet* seemed to be leaping out to me. I took it and flipped through it thinking that I would buy it in order to compare what the author had to say with our "healthy" diet of almost all raw foods. I also wanted to hear what the author had to say about cancer prevention. We had never heard of Michio Kushi or macrobiotics before.

On Monday morning, July 6, the biopsy proved the doctor to be correct. The diagnosis was a Stage III carcinoma of the urethra which had spread to the bladder. The doctor explained that this was a very rare cancer and extremely lethal. He felt it was most important to proceed quickly with all that was possible medically for the condition.

First, he set me up with the head radiologist who decided that a radium implant — the maximum for seven days — would be done on July 8. During my stay at Baylor Hospital, everyone was caring and efficient, but I was so sick with intense pain and nausea. Pain medication provided only temporary relief.

On July 17, my radiologist removed the implants and inserted a new catheter that remained in place for the next several weeks. After I left the hospital, the doctor checked me weekly and showed concern when, after six weeks, my strength had not returned. He and my urologist started planning and pressing me to have radical surgery by the following month.

I explained to the doctors that I was following a wonderful macrobiotic diet, but their reaction was that I was "too intelligent to believe that a diet or food had anything to do with cancer remission." Meanwhile, my husband found a macrobiotic center in Dallas and took cooking classes and bought supplies and books describing macrobiotic cancer recoveries. Thankfully, my husband, J. R., had always liked to cook and had been something of a health nut. So we embarked together on this new way of cooking, eating, and learning.

So it was only natural that I desired to go to Boston to meet with Michio Kushi. We called the Kushi Foundation and were able to meet with him on August 23. I was still quite weak and the unified message from most of my family and friends was to "put myself in the doctors' hands, since they knew best."

During our meeting, Mr. Kushi was cautiously optimistic. He felt that I would improve if I followed the macrobiotic recommendations, and suggested modifications in my diet along with home care preparations. He recommended walking for a half-hour each day, and suggested that I sing a happy song every day to keep my spirits up. He also emphasized chewing each mouthful at least fifty times.

Upon returning to Dallas, we followed Mr. Kushi's suggestions to the letter. We decided to delay the surgery and to see how things went. Gradually, my health and strength returned, and each visit to the doctor confirmed that the tumor was shrinking! In October, my doctor presented my case before the Dallas Board of Urologists. He felt that additional medical opinions would convince me of the urgency and necessity of radical surgery. I told him I appreciated his concern.

Shortly afterward, he called to report that all the doctors were of the opinion that surgery was critical to save my life, and that it must take place before December or else it would be too late. The reason I was so reluctant to have radical surgery was that it involved approximately sixteen hours of surgery, and seemingly one-fourth of my body would be cut out. Even with all this, my chances of surviving five years or longer were slim, and I was as concerned with the quality of life as I was with the quantity of years.

Early in November, we again went to see Mr. Kushi. He was delighted with my progress and was very optimistic about the chances for recovery. Again, we went home and continued very strictly on our healing diet. We prayed every step of the way and I also walked two miles daily and laughed and sang. I did not call the doctor again for he advised me not to until I had agreed to have surgery.

By the following June (1988), after returning home from Florida, I went to see the doctor. He was glad to see me and surprised to see how well and radiant I was. After conducting a cystoscopy, CT scans, x-rays, and blood work, he exclaimed that he was shocked and amazed that all the tests were clear — for now! He also said that my case would go into medical books, because no one with this condition had ever lived this long without radical surgery following the radium implant. I asked if he was just a little curious about what I had been doing during this time, but he just smiled and said, "Barbara, your body reacted extremely well to the radium implant and I know that you have great faith, but for sure, it is not that health diet you are on."

Upon leaving the doctor's office, J.R. and I were so excited that we jumped for joy and praised the Lord! There was rejoicing everywhere and with everyone. At a meeting of our macrobiotic group, everyone stood up and applauded and hugged us. The members of our church, as well as our family and friends who had prayed so faithfully for my healing, all rejoiced and shed many tears of thankfulness with us.

Since 1988, we have attended the annual Macrobiotic Summer Conference held in the Berkshire Mountains of Massachusetts. I have told my story in front of a large audience several times. A number of people with cancer who were attending the conference told me that my story encouraged and inspired them. These experiences have been overwhelming, and from that time telling my story to encourage others has become my ministry. In 1988, we started a cancer support group, the Lifeline, in order to help others. We started with only four people, and then it quickly grew to ten, and then twenty five, and beyond!

In April 1990, I told my story on a television show in Atlanta. Before going to Atlanta, I went to the doctor for an exam. He completed a cystoscopy and was amazed that the walls of my bladder were soft and pliable rather than rigid because of scar tissue. He said he saw no need for any further tests because it was clear that I had recovered. He stated that I was a "medical miracle."

In conclusion, the last three years have been some of the best years of my life. I feel deepest gratitude toward everyone and everything that contributed to my recovery: Michio Kushi, my expert doctors, the nutritionally balanced macrobiotic diet, physical exercise, and most importantly, the prayers and faith of my family and friends.

Sources: Correspondence with Barbara Lee, Dallas, Texas, January, 1991. Copyright © Barbara Lee.

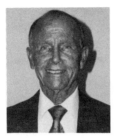

12.

J. R. Lee
Prostate Cancer

In early summer 1987, I began experiencing discomforting pains in my prostate area, especially when urinating which, incidentally, became more and more frequent. This caused me no undue concern, since for years, doctors had noted that my prostate was enlarged but posed no particular problem, so no medical attention had been recommended. As a former airline captain, I was required to pass a class one physical exam every six months for some thirty-three years and was otherwise always in excellent physical condition.

Attention was diverted from my condition, when in early July, my wife, Barbara, was diagnosed with cancer. Our prayers had led us to seek additional help in macrobiotics. In fact, I quickly completed classes in preparation and cooking of macrobiotic meals. That enabled me to cook for her, since she was completely incapacitated for a considerable time after the radium implant treatment and returning home from the hospital. As the people who make Morton salt say, "When it rains, it pours."

In August 1987, I had an alarming experience. Urination was

very restricted, accompanied by pain and slight traces of blood in my urine. Examination by a urologist revealed that I not only had a very enlarged prostate, but had a hard tumor on the right side. I inquired how it was possible to differentiate between the two. He replied, "There is no mistaking the two! Whereas the enlargement feels like flesh, the tumor has the feel of a large marble — bone-hard." Antibiotics were prescribed for an eight-day period. I told the doctor my wife and I were already on a special diet for our problems and would postpone a biopsy for the time being. He replied, "Well, they don't usually just go away."

In the meantime, my wife and I prayed more about this and were led to go to Boston to meet with Michio Kushi. I gave him my medical reports. He recommended special drinks to be taken twice a day for the first two weeks, and my routine was modified some for the next few weeks by phone. I read what I could on visualization and practiced it along with macrobiotics. It was evident that my condition was improving even though I continued to lose weight on the macrobiotic diet. My height is 5-10 1/2 and for some forty years my weight remained between 163 to 168, yet now my weight dropped to a low of 133 pounds before stabilizing and gradually increasing.

In late November 1987, I went back to the urologist. I had this good feeling all our prayers were being answered and was confident that the doctor was going to find that the tumor had shrunk quite a lot. But to be very candid, I could hardly believe I was hearing him correctly when he announced that he could find no trace of the tumor. I continued to improve and in December 1987, I went to the most renowned urologist in Dallas for a follow-up exam and sort of a second opinion. Quite a bit of enlargement remained but no trace of a tumor. It took almost a year for my weight to come back and level off at a steady 150. It is now February 1991, and I am seventy-one and in excellent health.

It is my hope and desire that this may be of some value to someone finding himself in a somewhat similar situation — to not panic, but calmly and methodically plot a course of action that he can have sufficient faith in, to in turn give him the hope necessary to enable his body, given proper nourishment and care, to heal itself.

Sources: Correspondence with J. R. Lee, February, 1991.

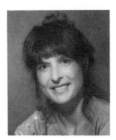

13.

Bonnie Kramer
Breast Cancer

In November 1980, Bonnie Kramer, a twenty-seven year old mother from Torrington, Connecticut, felt discomfort under her arm. She discovered a pea-sized ball that seemed to float when touched but was not overly concerned about it. She underwent a mammography the following February and the results were negative.

During the winter, the lump went through periods of increasing and decreasing size, and she started to experience constant pain in her left breast along with fatigue and a milky white discharge from the nipple. Her breasts were enlarged and tender. She also had an unusual number of colds and flu during the winter.

A biopsy in February 1982 revealed cancer, and soon afterward she entered Winsted Memorial Hospital in Connecticut for the removal of her left breast and several lymph nodes under her arm. She also began chemotherapy and was scheduled to undergo six weeks of radiation. The side effects were not severe, although she was irritable at times, lost some hair, and became nauseous after each treatment. She completed her treatments in March 1983, and was considered by her doctors to be free of cancer. However, periodic bone and liver scans were advised as a precaution. Feeling better, she took a job as a director of social services at a skilled nursing facility and helped raise funds for the American Cancer Society.

Three years later, in April 1986, while playing wiffle ball with her son, she felt a pull in her lower back. The pain continued off and on and by early 1987 had become unbearable. "The pain returned with a vengeance," she recalls. "It just would not go away, and the nurses at work became very concerned. The pain radiated in my face. With each menstrual cycle, I was bloated, suffering with intense cramps." She underwent a bone scan which revealed tumors on her pelvis and upper back. Her doctors advised radiation and aggressive chemotherapy. She was "numbed to speechlessness" at the news and "could hardly talk, and couldn't stop crying." As she recalls, "I had to deal with this; that's all I knew. I prayed for strength and guidance in the midst of all this drama. Then suddenly out of nowhere, it hit me! Honestly, just like that the answer came. I knew from my readings that more and more was coming out about nutrition and cancer. I remembered my sister telling me about an article she'd read several years before about a doctor whose cancer went into remission through a change in diet. It didn't seem relevant to me then, but suddenly, now it did. 'Oh my God,' I thought! 'That's what I need to do — find out more about this diet, but how?'"

Her friend went to a local health food store and bought a copy of Michio Kushi's *The Macrobiotic Way* for her to read. Bonnie found it completely logical but overwhelming. She went to the health food store and bought staple foods and stopped eating meat, sugar, and dairy food. She also underwent radiation therapy and a hysterectomy and after recovering from surgery decided to attend the Macrobiotic Way of Life Seminar presented by the Kushi Institute.

Bonnie supplemented her practice of macrobiotics by taking weekly cooking classes with Sarah Lapenta, a K.I. cooking teacher who lived nearby. By May 1987, a blood test revealed that her enzyme levels had returned to normal. A bone scan in September showed that the tumors had greatly decreased in size. A friend who worked in the radiation unit at the hospital told her that she had never seen a report like that before. In September 1988, another bone scan revealed the presence of scar tissue but no tumors. Her doctor told her that her remission might have been due to the surgery and radiation but that macrobiotics may have also helped her. By August 1988, a bone scan produced a totally normal result, with no tumors or scar tissue. Her doctor was now very impressed and fully supportive of her macrobiotic lifestyle.

Bonnie describes her macrobiotic experience: "I noticed immediate changes in myself and my son, Ben, who joined in my meals for the first summer. Our allergies seemed to disappear and Ben no longer got strep throat. We felt stronger, energetic, more organized, and very well. I had good spirits and stable moods. As my confidence increased, so did the sense of inner peace. I loved feeling at one with nature, at one with God."

Bonnie is now preparing to open a macrobiotic center in her area. She believes that "happiness is real only if it can be shared with others." She would like to help people in her area through classes, food, and guidance. She has dedicated herself to realizing one peaceful world and is grateful to have found a way to "help make this concept a reality."

Source: "A Mother Heals Breast Cancer: Change in Diet Aids Remission of Tumors and Metatases to the Bone," *One Peaceful World* Newsletter, Becket, Massachusetts, Spring, 1990.

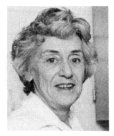

14.

Virginia Brown
Malignant Melanoma

In August 1978, Virginia Brown, a fifty-six year old mother and registered nurse from Tunbridge, Vermont, noticed a black mole on her arm that kept getting bigger and blacker. She had lost a lot of weight and felt very dull mentally. Doctors at Vermont Medical Center in Burlington performed a biopsy and discovered that she had an advanced case of malignant melanoma (Stage IV). The physicians told her that without surgery she could expect to live only six months. "Even though I had been trained and practiced in the medical profession for years," she later recalled, "I could not go along with surgery. I had professed alternatives for years but did not really practice them."

At home, her son and daughter-in-law encouraged her to try macrobiotics, and shortly thereafter she attended the East West Foundation's annual cancer conference, meeting that year in Amherst, Massachusetts. At the conference she listened to fifteen cancer patients discuss their experiences on the diet and was impressed with their accounts.

Prior to that time she had followed the standard American way of eating, high in refined foods and fat, especially animal fat from dairy foods, beef, poultry, and fish. At the time she started the diet, she was so sick that she could hardly make it upstairs and slept most of the day. After three weeks eating the new food, which her children prepared for her, she experienced a change in her energy level, attitude, and mental clarity. "I was a new person; I could get up and walk around."

In September she went to Boston to see Michio Kushi, and he made more specific dietary recommendations and advised her to study cooking. With the support of her family, she adhered faithfully to the diet, supplemented by yoga, prayer and meditation, and a two-mile walk each morning after breakfast.

In 1979, it became apparent that Virginia had overcome her condition, and medical exams subsequently confirmed her recovery. After restoring her health, Virginia went on to study at the Kushi Institute and to work as a nurse in the macrobiotic health program that was started at the Lemuel Shattuck Hospital in Boston, promoting a more natural way of living among other medical professionals and patients. In 1984, her story was published by Japan Publications in the book *Macrobiotic Miracle: How a Vermont Family Overcame Cancer.*

Sources: "Malignant Melanoma, Stage IV," in *Cancer and Diet* (East West Foundation, 1980); interview with Alex Jack, September 30, 1982; Virginia Brown, with Susan Stayman, *Macrobiotic Miracle: How a Vermont Family Overcame Cancer* (Japan Publications, 1984).

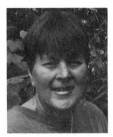

15.

Magdaline Cronley
Breast and Lung Cancer

My name is Magdaline Cronley and I live in the easternmost town on Long Island, Montauk, with my husband Bob and daughter Jennifer. I am forty-seven years old and was brought up on what is known as the American diet. I consumed large quantities of meat, dairy products, sugar, frozen foods, and last, but not least, fast foods. I smoked cigarettes for over thirty years. Throughout my life I suffered with colds, flu, sinus problems, kidney infections, cysts, and weight problems.

In August 1984, I was diagnosed as having breast and lung cancer that had spread to various bones in my body. The prognosis was that I had two months to live as the cancer was deemed terminal and inoperable. I immediately began chemotherapy, which resulted in every hair on my body falling out and my not being able to keep down any food. When I wasn't vomiting, I was thinking about it. This way of life continued for a month, resulting in my body becoming weaker daily.

In September, a woman named Joanne Kushi (formerly Joanne Collette), lent my husband a copy of *The Cancer Prevention Diet* by Michio Kushi. That book was the ray of sunshine I had been waiting for. It became my Bible. I carried it around with me. It was on the night table next to my bed, in case I needed to look something up during the night. I started to see that if I ate the American diet I would feel worse and vomit, as some of the additives in food and cosmetics were the same as those in my chemotherapy treatments. If I would have a visitor who perhaps had on perfume or aftershave lotion containing these additives, I would say hello and have to excuse myself to go throw up.

As soon as I started to cook and eat miso soup, brown rice, and steamed vegetables, I began to feel better and stronger and the vomiting subsided. I started to cook in my wheelchair. Each day I was getting stronger. My doctor had wanted to give me two years of chemotherapy, which was twenty-two months longer than I was expected to live. He believed that without chemotherapy I would not survive. I continued chemotherapy for an additional six months and prepared special dishes to rebuild my blood after each treatment.

I also had to deal with the cause of my cancer. I had to accept that smoking for thirty years had contributed to my lung cancer, and that eating a diet high in dairy products had most likely contributed to my breast cancer. Once I realized that I had helped my body get into this situation, I also realized that I could turn this illness into a blessing and allow God to heal me. I now had the ways and means to change my condition.

During January 1985, I started to call in well for my chemotherapy treatments. I would feel so great that I didn't want to go for a treatment and spoil things, for example, by starting to vomit and losing my hair. I had lost every hair on my body three times. I also grew back every hair three times with the help of good food. We also went to Florida for a vacation and walked on the beach, went into the salt water, ate good macrobiotic meals, and were thankful for what we had.

In March 1985, I went into the hospital for a blood transfusion after having been given too much chemotherapy. My doctor said that if I didn't have the transfusion, I would be in serious trouble if I came in contact with anyone carrying any germ that my immune system was unable to neutralize. In other words, my immune system was extremely weak. I realized that after the many X-rays, scans, and chemotherapy my body had become toxic and had it not been for miso, sea vegetables, brown rice and vegetables, I would probably not have survived.

I started taking cooking classes and attending macrobiotic conferences and also went to the Kushi Institute in Becket, Massachusetts. I feel very fortunate to have been taught by the best teachers in the world. I realized that sharing had a great deal to do with my recovery. Our friend, Joanne, shared her knowledge and book with me, which resulted in my being able to heal myself. I was told that once you heal yourself, like it or not, you become a healer. I have since helped anyone who would listen and even sometimes those who weren't listening.

I teach cooking classes in our little hamlet of Montauk and nearby. To me, macrobiotics is not to be kept in a treasure chest but shared with whomever needs and wants to learn about it. Six years after my struggle with terminal cancer, I am alive and well, and thanking God for the opportunity to help others just as I was helped.

Source: Correspondence with Magdaline Cronley, Montauk, New York, August, 1990.

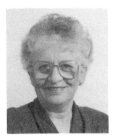

16.

Anne Kramer
Breast Cancer

In February 1986, I was diagnosed with breast cancer. I underwent a modified radical mastectomy of my left breast. Four out of twelve lymph nodes were found to have metatastic carcinoma, plus microscopic tumor emboli were present within small auxillary blood vessels. My oncologist recommended chemotherapy for a year, possibly longer. A second opinion from another oncologist was the same — a year or more of chemotherapy. He suggested that I probably had several thousand cancer cells floating around in my bloodstream. It wasn't a happy picture. Also, a routine hospital blood test revealed my cholesterol level to be 243.

While I was healing from the mastectomy, I started reading cancer research reports of studies relating high fat content diets to breast cancer. One such study of Japanese women eating traditional Japanese foods showed a much lower incidence of breast cancer and a lower recurrence rate when compared to Western women eating standard American high-fat foods. I knew I needed to get on a low-fat diet, but I had no energy to search for a traditional Japanese diet. I was weak from chemotherapy. My doctor had put me on Coopers' regimen. I also took Tamoxifin because the receptor test had been slightly positive. Three months into difficult chemotherapy treatments, a friend told me about a macrobiotic diet. I sent for the book *The Cancer-Prevention Diet* by Michio Kushi. I read the book and immediately started cooking meals recommended for my illness. I knew this macrobiotic diet was what I was looking for. I believed it would help me heal myself of breast cancer. My feelings of helplessness went away. I became more optimistic about the outcome of my disease.

It was not easy to shop and cook the new strange foods, especially since I had absolutely no energy and felt sick and nauseated much of the time — side effects of the chemotherapy treatments. At least I didn't have to worry about getting hair in the food — I didn't have any left on my head! I believed in this new diet and followed the directions religiously. Aveline Kushi's peaceful recipes made me feel calm and in charge of my getting well. I also read the book by the Simontons, *Getting Well Again*, and did the recommended visualization exercises three times a day.

After two months on the diet, I had a repeat mammogram on my right breast. The doctor had warned me of the possibility of new tumors where calcification spots had been found. I was anxious. The mammograms revealed that the calcification spots were gone! The calcification spots found six months earlier were gone! I was elated.

In September 1986, I made up my mind to stop chemotherapy. My oncologist didn't like or agree with my decision and told me I should stay on chemotherapy for another six months or longer. My mind rebelled at the thought of another six months of that poison. On several occasions the doctor couldn't perform chemotherapy treatments on me because my white blood cells were dangerously low. I promised my body I would not undergo any further chemotherapy treatments.

Later that fall I met Bonnie Breidenbach, a macrobiotic teacher in the Detroit area. She fine-tuned the diet for me. Bonnie also told me about a doctor who had group therapy for cancer patients. I attended the group sessions for awhile. To share feelings with other people who had cancer and were living the macrobiotic way of life was very encouraging and supportive.

It is now almost five years later and I am healthy. Repeated mammograms, bone scans, chest x-rays, and blood tests show no trace of cancer. I am sixty-one years old, my cholesterol reading is 170, and I have enrolled in the Kushi Institute Extension Program in Cleveland to learn more about macrobiotics. I enjoy the program and I'm enjoying life. I am grateful that my husband is supportive and went on the diet with me from the start. I am also grateful that my child, grandchildren, and eighty-nine year old mother are benefiting from this diet as well.

I am also thankful to God for giving me illness and health to help me appreciate life.

Source: Correspondence with Anne Kramer, Washington, Michigan, January, 1991.

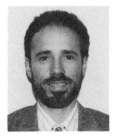

17.

Brian Bonaventura
Brain Tumor

My name is Brian Bonaventura from Columbus, Ohio, and I'm thirty-seven years old. I work in the automotive industry and I have recovered from two brain tumors with the help of macrobiotics and spiritual growth. This is my story.

My diet before cancer was the standard American diet — red meat, sweets, fried food, coffee and sodas. I had also repressed my emotions for many years and had never been truly happy, although my general health was all right. I had been suffering flu-like symptoms for several months when in September 1983, I suffered from a seizure at work. I was diagnosed as having a benign brain tumor the size of a small orange in the right frontal lobe of my brain. I had surgery immediately and completely recovered with no paralysis.

After considering differing opinions between my radiologist and oncologist as to whether or not I should have radiation and/or chemotherapy treatments, I finally agreed with the radiologist that because of my young age — twenty-nine at the time — and the fact that two of the three reports from pathologists said the tumor was benign, I could forego chemotherapy at this time. My neurosurgeon agreed but felt I should begin radiation right away. I decided not to and began to try and put my life together again by trying to save my struggling marriage and overcome my increasing fear of crowds. Less than a year later, I began having panic attacks at work and started taking tranquilizers to be able to cope with work and home. Looking back, I now realize this was not a good sign. My panic attacks stopped as soon as I began using tranquilizers, but I severely disturbed my normal sleep and dream patterns for the four years I was taking them. I was also adversely affected by the strong, humid heat of Ohio summers and avoided activity as much as possible during this time. After another CT scan in the fall of 1984, I decided to change doctors. My test results were all normal, but my new doctor advised me to avoid fried foods and decrease my meat consumption, as the triglyceride levels in my blood were elevated. This was the first advice I had received from a doctor about changing my diet.

Both 1985 and 1986 passed without any major changes in my physical condition. I was having yearly CT scans which were normal, and by that time, had been advised by my doctor to also cut back on dairy products. As my emotional life became more and more stressful, I began craving oily, fatty foods and went through periods of dieting and binging. I began a program of physical conditioning in 1984 to overcome some gain in weight that had begun to be a problem. Although the physical conditioning and bicycle training helped me somewhat, my dietary habits slipped back to the same old patterns of high amounts of fat and sugar again, and my marriage was worse off than ever. The summer heat had become intolerable again, and by this time the tranquilizers I had been taking all this time were becoming ineffective. I began consuming alcohol to deal with my increasing emotional depressions.

I finally ended my marriage in 1988. That year, I had a test called an MRI (Magnetic Resonance Imaging) that revealed another tumor in the same place of my brain. After another surgery and another complete recovery, my neurosurgeon emphatically recommended radiation treatments, as he was sure the second tumor was malignant. Physically, I once expected modern medicine to take away all of my troubles. Now after going through two brain tumors and two major surgeries within the space of five years, I began to see that for me, this wasn't going to be the case. As my consciousness changed, I feel now it was no coincidence that my sister-in-law gave me a copy of Dr. Anthony Sattilaro's book *Recalled By Life* while I was recovering from my second surgery. After weighing my options, I decided enthusiastically to give macrobiotics a try. I couldn't put the book down and felt it made complete sense, reviewing my past. As soon as I got out of the hospital, I located the nearest health food co-op and began eating as close to the macrobiotic diet as I knew how, while reading all I could. After a meeting with Michio, I followed his suggestions very closely for many months.

My health has improved dramatically in three years. Emotionally, I'm much more stable than I ever have been and no longer take tranquilizers as I haven't had a panic attack in years. I use alcohol very rarely now and never because I'm depressed. Since starting macrobiotics, I hardly ever get depressed! I also have lost the cravings I once had for fatty foods because I eat a very balanced diet. After following Michio's recommendation to use a poultice over the place on my head where the surgery was, I have lost a persistent ringing in my right ear and feel confident that I have overcome my last encounter with brain tumors.

I am an avid snow and water-skier, and my physical health has never been better. I am now very active in the macrobiotic community of Columbus and have also decided to eventually become a macrobiotic counselor. My life has shown me that disease manifests itself mentally long before it shows up on a CT scan. I believe diet and emotions are the foundation to health or disease. Now I allow my life to be my prognosis. A macrobiotic diet has given me that freedom. If one has the courage, one's dream can become a reality. Life, for me, has never been more fulfilling. I no longer rely on the medical profession for answers, only assistance. I believe the only real cure for cancer lies in us finding the truth behind our disease, within ourselves, and in our universe. Thank you, macrobiotics, for another chance at life!

Source: Correspondence with Brian Bonaventura, Columbus, Ohio, April, 1991.

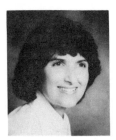

18.

Elaine Nussbaum
Uterine Cancer

In April 1980, I was diagnosed with uterine cancer. It was a mixed tumor, a carcinosarcoma, and it was embedded in the muscle of the lining of the connective tissue of my uterus. I was treated with external and internal radiation, oral and intravenous chemotherapy, and hormone therapy. In August 1980, I had a radical hysterectomy. I continued to take chemotherapy.

In May 1982, I started having pain in my lower back, which was diagnosed as a compression fracture. Despite strong medication, the pain got progressively worse. I could neither sit nor lie down. In August, after a few days of standing up all day and night, sleeping only on my husband's shoulder in a standing position, I consulted an orthopedist. The orthopedist confirmed the compression fracture and noted that I also had a partially collapsed vertebrae. In order to prevent a total collapse of my backbone, I was put into a brace which extended from below my chest to below my pelvis and wrapped around my back. I wore the brace all day and night.

The pain got worse and spread to my legs. When I could no

longer stand, I was placed in a recliner chair, where I stayed in a semi-reclining position taking strong painkillers around the clock. Nothing stopped the pain.

In September, I was carried back to the hospital for more diagnostic procedures. These tests showed that, in addition to the collapsed backbone, I had cancer on my lumbar spine, cancer on my thoracic spine, and multiple metastatic deposits in both lungs.

I was given radiation again, then chemotherapy, then more radiation, then more chemotherapy. The protocol for me was for ten cycles of chemotherapy, given at three- to four-week intervals. Each treatment required an overnight stay in the hospital. I was tired, weak, nauseous, and in pain.

Toward the end of January 1983, after four cycles of chemotherapy, I cut my finger on an envelope. Because my blood levels were so depressed from the chemotherapy, I was unable to fight the infection that set in. The paper-cut resulted in a ten-day hospital stay, which included massive doses of intravenous antibiotics, four blood transfusions, and three days in isolation. The doctors then decided that the chemotherapy I was getting was too strong for me; I would be put on something less toxic.

Diagnostic procedures performed during the hospital stay showed unchanged metastatic cancer in both my lungs and increased activity and progression of the cancer in my spine.

It was then that I realized that conventional medicine was not helping me, and I began to consider an alternative. I chose macrobiotics based mostly on my reading about other people who had healed themselves with this approach. Particularly inspiring was Dr. Sattilaro's story. I felt that if he could recover his health, I could too.

In February 1983, I began to practice macrobiotics. I completely eliminated from my diet all meat, poultry, eggs, fish, dairy food, sugar, and fruit. I reduced to zero the thirty-eight pills I was taking every day. I decided to stop all chemotherapy, hormone therapy, antibiotics, and vitamin supplements. I started to eat brown rice and cooked vegetables.

I began macrobiotics in a hospital bed, a wheelchair, a brace, and in pain. The pain gradually subsided, and I never took another painkiller. After a short time, I was able to take a few steps with the help of a walker. I practiced walking with the walker, then with two canes, then with one cane. In April, a urinary problem that had plagued me for three years (a result of the original radiation) disappeared. In mid-May I took off the brace. On May 22, I walked for the first time all by myself.

In June, I put away my wig; my hair, which had all fallen out from the chemotherapy, had grown back enough to be presentable. I returned the hospital bed. I started driving again. I resumed my studies towards my master's degree in nutrition. Within six months I had changed from a sick, depressed, pill popping invalid, to a happy, optimistic, and very, very grateful pain-free person.

It is now eight years that I have been living the macrobiotic way, and I continue to enjoy good health. I completed the Master's of Science degree in nutrition; my thesis was on the macrobiotic approach to cancer. I continue to study, practice, and teach macrobiotics. I have an active counseling practice, and I also offer macrobiotic cooking classes. My book entitled *Recovery: From Cancer to Health through Macrobiotics* (Japan Publications, 1986) has inspired thousands of people to improve their health with macrobiotics.

Some important factors in my recovery have included accurate practice of macrobiotic recommendations (no cheating); regular visits with a macrobiotic teacher; shiatsu massage; love and support from family and friends; a lot of prayer; and a positive and optimistic attitude. My experiences, both personal and professional, have shown me some of the wonderful changes that can occur when living the macrobiotic way.

Source: Correspondence with Elaine Nussbaum, West Orange, New Jersey, November, 1990.

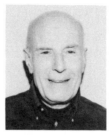

19.

Herb Walley
Prostate Cancer

When I was in my early forties, I suffered severe blockage of the urinary tract which necessitated a transurethral operation on my enlarged prostate. Subsequent multiple adhesions required reaming, stretching, and splitting of the tube. This apparently caused the tumor to develop. By the time I reached my sixties this growth had become malignant. My urologist, believing he had caught it soon enough to hold it in abeyance by the use of hormones, instead of a major operation, placed me on a regimen of rather heavy doses of stilbesterol, a female hormone. This was at about age sixty-three. Stilbesterol is one drug that so-called "female impersonators" use to change their physique, eliminate body hair, and develop full breasts. The side effects are pretty awful for a man who wants to remain masculine.

Some of the more depressing transformations are breast and nipple enlargement with extreme tenderness, fluid retention throughout the body — the legs in particular — with resulting inconvenience of hourly toilet trips, both day and night. Also, loss of fingernail substance results in painful split and torn nails. There are many other less obvious effects which are equally annoying.

After many visits to the urologist, with constant reminders to take my daily dosage for the rest of my life, I finally inveighed him to reduce the hormone strength by half. However, this didn't help appreciably.

As I approached age sixty-eight, with the tumor still testing malignant, a good friend and neighbor was diagnosed as having cancer of the prostate. His wife, a novelist, was given a copy of *Recalled By Life* by her publisher. After reading it, they pursued the macrobiotic diet. Once read, the book was given to me. As I entered my seventieth year this book offered a possible solution to my discomfort. A meeting with a macrobiotic teacher at the Kushi Institute provided me with specific guidelines for my condition. After one month I felt more alive and much less depressed. I stopped taking all medications and vitamins and made monthly visits to my general practitioner for checkups. I made several more visits to the Kushi Institute for dietary adjustments. I also lost sixty-five pounds of old fat from all over my body.

Ten macrobiotic months later, I returned to my doctor to report on what I had accomplished. Very upset, he advised me that "If the results of the tests showed any signs of cancer, you must immediately start major curative measures (chemotherapy). If the tests showed no cancer, then just keep on doing whatever you're doing." He had no knowledge of, or desire to learn about, macrobiotics. All tests came back negative. To be certain, I checked into the Dana Farber Cancer Research Center. After many tests and a complete bone scan, I was assured that I was "clean."

If you have no medical reason to consider macrobiotics, but would like a rewarding old age with health and happiness, you can gradually adopt a new way of eating. Your body will accept the change graciously. If medically necessary, first make certain that you have support at home, then seek out qualified help. Attend a program such as the Macrobiotic Residential Seminar presented at the Kushi Institute of the Berkshires that offers a peaceful and happy atmosphere while you are learning to cook and live the macrobiotic way. Bring your family support person with you, if possible, for a week or so of cooking instruction and practice. Follow the diet carefully when you return home and keep in contact with a macrobiotic teacher for fine-tuning and adjustments. At all times keep a positive mental attitude and use mental imagery to overcome your illness.

Those of you who can accept a change in lifestyle will find many rewards in an exciting and beautiful future. If you can't accept changes, at least reduce your consumption of red meats, chemically contaminated poultry, sugar, refined table salt, and junk foods. Remember that basically no diet will cure; it can only cleanse the body of toxins and fats. Then mental attitude and imagery can work together to awaken the body's immune system to overcome the disease. The combination of these two factors in a relaxing environment almost invariably leads to better health.

As of November 1990, I am almost seventy-seven years old. I am still "clean" with almost unlimited energy. I can eat all I want without gaining weight, and look forward to another twenty or thirty years of excitement and happiness.

Source: *The Macrobiotic Experience*, newsletter published by Herb and Virginia Walley, Newton, Massachusetts, November, 1990.

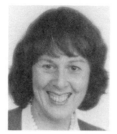

20.

Diane Silver Hassell
Thyroid Cancer*

As a child, I was fed a balanced diet (according to modern under-standing) and given many vitamin supplements as I grew up. I was sick fairly often as a child; I recall colds, earaches, that kind of thing. I had a very bad case of pneumonia when I was two years old and was given a sulfa drug, which was then in its primitive stages. I had tonsils and adenoids removed at the age of four. The adenoids grew back, and when I was ten they were removed again by experimental radium treatment.

I had to push myself very hard to keep up with the other students at school in athletics, but I became a very good swimmer. I also led a very active social life. I was teaching school full-time by the time I was nineteen and was married at twenty. In 1960, when I was twenty-three, a routine examination turned up a very large dark,

*I claim no "cancer cure" in strictly medical terms because I had a thyroidectomy and subsequent replacement therapy. However, as my account indicates, my uterine fibroids spontaneously disappeared; my general health improved markedly; and I have had no new lymph node involvement or other "bumps or lumps" since beginning a macrobiotic diet in 1975.

fast-growing mole on my forehead.   It was removed and diagnosed as a melanoma.

In 1969, a large fibroid tumor was removed from my uterus. Before that operation, my blood count was down to 30; I hemorrhaged in the hospital, had a cardiac arrest, and was pronounced dead. I left my body but then decided to return to life in order to raise my children. In early 1971, a tumor was found in a lymph node on my neck. I was concerned about melanoma and was relieved when the diagnosis was papillary and follicular carcinoma of the thyroid. My doctor then made two quick moves. He looked up the slides of the pathology report of my melanoma and showed them to a pathologist friend, who declared that to be a somewhat questionable diagnosis. He also sent me off for the removal of my thyroid gland and many other lymph nodes in my neck, which proved malignant.

In the years between 1957 and 1971, several other conditions had troubled me. Every few months I would have severe painful cystitis and would be treated with some form of sulfa. I had frequent recurring bouts of pneumonia, for which I received antibiotics regularly. I had a painful troublesome diaphragmatic hernia. I was advised to sleep in a sitting position. I had premenstrual tension, edema, and severe menstrual cramps. I took diuretics and birth control pills.

Between 1971 and 1975, a few more bumps were biopsied from my back and breast, but they were all benign. I was feeling tired and draggy most of the time. I put on forty-five extra pounds. My bladder condition and diaphragmatic hernia were troubling me, and I kept getting colds and pneumonia. I had irregular Pap smear tests for three years. I was checked, x-rayed, and scanned for cancer at regular intervals.

By the fall of 1975, I was really sick! My endocrinologist was very concerned. He decided on a complete series of tests and x-rays for me. After a cystoscopic examination, a urologist declared that I would have to take sulfa the rest of my life because there was a stricture in my urethra that was causing chronic infection.

I had two intravenous pyelograms which turned up a finding, suspicions of a malignancy on one of my kidneys. Upper and lower gastrointestinal series and scans for cancer showed nothing conclusive. My cholesterol was high, too, but these tests offered no real answers to the constant fatigue and frequent pneumonia bouts. My endocrinologist thought that I had better stop taking the birth control pill. My gynecologist suggested a change of pill but advised that I should continue that medication because I had growing fibroid tumors that would grow out of control if I stopped.

In late October 1975, I was sick in bed with pneumonia and again on antibiotics. I felt a new lymph node growing on the back of my neck. I rested for weeks with no improvement at all. This sickness seemed very different: I was not getting any better and my physicians were stumped.

One day I received a phone call from a pleasant young man named Alan Ginsberg, phoning to deliver regards from a mutual friend in New York. When he heard my gasping and coughing, he remarked, "You sound sick." "Yes, I have pneumonia," I rasped. "What are you eating?" Well, in all my thirty-eight years of life, no physician had ever asked what I was eating.

I told Alan I was eating some cottage cheese, salad, lots of grapefruit and orange juice "because I need fluids." He asked me if I had considered that there were nine to twelve grapefruits in the two or three glasses of juice I was having every day; that grapefruits grow in hot climates — "That this is November and you are in Toronto in the winter and it is getting cold, and furthermore, cottage cheese and all dairy foods create mucus in the body, and you don't need any more mucus!" Was he some kind of nut, I wondered? Or was he making sense?

Was it possible that what I ate could really make a difference in how I felt? I was really very anxious to get well, so I decided to listen. He asked me if I had any whole grains in the house; I only had oatmeal. He advised me to eat just oatmeal, with no milk or sugar on it, for several days and he would call back. I was terribly skeptical; but after a few days of just oatmeal I was out of bed, feeling better and ready to listen to what Alan had to say.

He instructed me in the basics of macrobiotics and I began to read. He also offered treatments to get my energy moving. After a few months I was strong enough to begin very simple exercise and to take short walks again. I was still skeptical but I was determined to give it a wholehearted try.

I stopped all medication except the birth control pill and the Synthoid. The bladder infection never returned. At the end of December 1975, Michio Kushi came to lecture in Toronto and reaffirmed for me everything Alan had said. He amazed me because he understood my condition simply by looking at my face.

Mr. Kushi thought that I was still cancerous and suggested a list of foods to eat and those to avoid. In February, I informed my gynecologist that I was stopping the birth control pill. He assured me that I would be back for a hysterectomy very shortly because the fibroids would grow wildly. The following year at my regular checkup he reported that the fibroids had disappeared and that I was in better shape than I had been for years. My Pap smear was normal and has remained so. Since then my diaphragmatic hernia has caused no further trouble; my menstrual periods come and go without pain, swelling, or tension at all. I do not get pneumonia any more, although I occasionally cough up phlegm without any sick feeling. There have been no further lumps or bumps. Even the varicose veins in my legs have disappeared.

Last winter, I took up cross-country skiing and ice skating again. I used to feel chilled all winter. Now I find pleasure at being outdoors in the cold. My attitude and my body have changed drastically; my entire life has changed for the better.

When Edward Esko telephoned to request permission to reprint the speech I had given at the 1978 Macrobiotic Summer Conference, I was pleased. However, I wanted to update the story because the past thirteen years since 1978 have been so full of challenges and changes for me and I have learned so much more about healing myself, while continuing macrobiotic eating.

I decided to leave the original speech unchanged because it is an honest and joyous picture of how I felt after three years of macrobiotic practice. My addendum follows.

Between 1978 and the end of 1981, I ran a successful macrobiotic center in my home with hundreds of people attending cooking classes and dinners each week and monthly seminars with macrobiotic teachers from the U.S. I'd like to mention just a few of the many things I learned from these visiting lecturers: to express my gratitude for difficulties daily and to enjoy growing and developing myself through my problems, to do physical exercises to improve my posture and energy and to engage in self-reflection every day as an important part of my macrobiotic practice.

I remarried in 1981 and welcomed the challenges of a new relationship and of the integration of a large family of three stepsons and my own two sons. I continued to work as a lifestyle counselor and teacher in my husband's holistic medical clinic, drawing on my thirty years of school teaching experience and my self-healing studies. I earned a brown belt in karate. My health remained good and I handled any small problems with macrobiotic remedies such as healing foods, compresses, etc.

I think that every time we get stuck or rigid in our beliefs, something happens to shake us up. I believed firmly that those with sufficient will could heal themselves with macrobiotic practice, even if they had to drag themselves to the stove as I had done at first. I think I was due for a lesson and it came in early 1989.

I became badly chilled while practicing karate outdoors at our vacation home in northern Ontario. Annoyed with myself for feeling so exhausted and giving in to the flu or perhaps the pneumonia that ensued, I continued to push myself to exercise hard. I developed myocarditis, pericarditis and pneumonitis and I collapsed. What followed was a combination of Western medical diagnostic methods, massage lovingly given by my husband, sons, stepsons and practitioner friends, wonderful macrobiotic foods and remedies prepared by caring colleagues and herbal and homeopathic remedies as well. I was in a hospital bed at home, on oxygen for about three weeks. I recovered slowly for almost a year, enough time to recognize that I couldn't possibly have survived without a lot of help and that there was value, after all, in Western medical support. I also realized more than ever before, that the emotional and spiritual difficulties that caused so much sickness in my early life would surely make me sick again if I didn't make real changes.

I began to practice yoga and Reiki, still too weak for much karate. I attended personal growth seminars and meditated daily. A huge outpouring of love from family, colleagues and friends surrounded me, broke down my rigidity and led me to more gentleness, kindness and respect for myself and others. My deep inner sadness faded and courage took its place as my lungs healed.

However, less physical activity, more relaxation and too much good macrobiotic food led to a startling increase in weight until I had almost reached my pre-macrobiotic state of tubbiness. I felt heavy and tired a lot of the time. Expressions like "over the hill" and "past her prime" started to seem relevant.

My most recent lesson has come from the little book by Namboku Mizuno called *Food Governs Your Destiny*, translated from Japanese by Aveline and Michio Kushi and Alex Jack. Following its principles of eating only at regular times, eating only if hungry and eating less than one wants, I've lost ten pounds in the last month and, already, I have more energy and feel more control over my life than I can ever remember.

In conclusion, in my opinion, macrobiotic eating is a necessary first step in giving our bodies a chance to heal. But this first step must be followed by macrobiotic living which includes seven levels: physical, sensory, psychological, mental, social, philosophical and spiritual — meaning a total acceptance of all life as it is. I believe that a "cure" based on food alone cannot carry us for more than a few years.

Also, it seems to me that perfect health would not be a total absence of all physical or emotional problems but rather a strong flexible body and mind which incorporate small problems from time to time in order to adjust and make balance.

For me, there will doubtless be more challenges — physical, emotional and spiritual — but whatever happens and wherever I find myself, I plan to enjoy it.

Sources: Diane Silver Hassell, "Thyroid Cancer, Fibroid Tumors," in Michio Kushi, *Cancer and Heart Disease: The Macrobiotic Approach*, Japan Publications, 1982; correspondence with Diane Silver Hassell, Richmond Hill, Ontario, April, 1991.

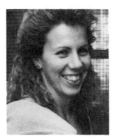

21.

Christina Pirello
Leukemia

My mother and I were very close. When she was diagnosed with colon cancer in 1982, I thought nothing worse could happen. Then, when she died in 1984, at forty-nine years of age, my life was rocked to the core. Her illness and death, ironically, set me on the path I follow today.

I watched as conventional methods of treatment hastened her deterioration. Watching her suffer more with each treatment strengthened my convictions to seek out alternative treatments should I ever find myself in a similar situation. I had absolutely no idea what that meant, but I knew that I could never go through a similar ordeal. Interestingly, one of her doctors mentioned macrobiotics to me, but it was too late for her, and I forgot all about it.

My maternal family history is checkered with diabetes, cancer, and anemia, so it was no surprise when, as a child, I was diagnosed with Mediterranean anemia. Every female member of my family was plagued with this disease.

Throughout my teenage years, I seemed relatively healthy, but always had the hardest time healing cuts and scratches. Bruises seemed to appear from nowhere. Stamina was always a problem as well. My menstrual cycle was irregular and so doctors began hormone treatments which would last for over fifteen years.

At the age of fourteen, I decided to become a vegetarian (whatever that means). I continued to eat lots of dairy, sugar, and refined foods. After my mother died, my fatigue worsened. I thought it was just an accumulation of exhaustion from over two years of taking care of her and dealing with my grief. I felt drained all the time. As the months after her death wore on, it seemed that my condition worsened — bruises were appearing everywhere; I felt as though my insides were on fire.

Finally, after five months of living in this manner, I decided that a fresh start would be what I needed. So I packed up and left Florida and moved North to Philadelphia. As I settled into my new surroundings, my health continued to worsen. Bruises appeared from nowhere; minor scratches became infected and would not heal; and I was exhausted. I finally decided to see a doctor, who, after a battery of tests, referred me to a hemotologist/oncologist. I was put through every test they could think of, after which they came up with the diagnosis of chronic myelocytic leukemia.

So here I was, twenty-seven years old, sitting in a room with five hemotologists recounting my options — as they saw them. With a lymphocyte count as high as mine, they really did not see a sunny future for me. However, they did want to propose experimental chemotherapy and a possible bone marrow transplant. When I questioned them as to a time frame, their response was not encouraging — three months to live with no treatment, and six months to a year with treatment. It seemed to me that the only guarantee I could get from them was that I would lose my hair and feel lousy for the time I had left. All I could think of was what my mother went through. I said I needed a few days to digest all of this. I knew I would never go back there.

For about a week, I walked around in a daze. Here I was, faced with this crisis, in a new city, with nowhere to turn. Finally I spoke to a friend at work and told him everything. I told him that my plan was to return to Europe and live there until the end came. He suggested that before I do anything quite that drastic, that I meet a friend of his who ate this strange diet that was supposed to help people recover from diseases like cancer. I figured I had nothing to lose and agreed.

That weekend I was introduced to Robert Pirello, who had been practicing macrobiotics for eight years, and my life was changed forever.

Bob was great. He listened to all my fears and finally agreed to help me as much as he could. The next day, we went shopping. I watched as Bob loaded up my cart with all these unfamiliar foods. I couldn't even pronounce the names I was going to cook and eat them? But, then again, I thought, I had always loved a challenge. What bigger challenge than seeing if I could heal my own illness?

We went back to my apartment and Bob cleaned out my cupboards — throwing away all the old foods and replacing them with this new food. As I watched, I began to get really scared — a challenge was one thing, but this was my life. If I messed this up, there were no second chances. As Bob left, he handed me *The Cancer-Prevention Diet* by Michio Kushi, telling me to read and cook. I read all night.

We met for lunch every day. Bob brought rice balls or leftovers from his own dinner. (Although I was a great conventional cook, my macrobiotic cooking was terrible then.) We talked and talked and I read and read. After a few weeks, I had lost weight and had more energy. Then I had a blood test — my lymphocyte count had worsened. Now I was scared. Even macrobiotics wasn't working. I felt hopeless. But, with Bob's encouragement, I persevered. I began to cook in earnest. It suddenly occurred to me that only I could make me well. Bob wanted me to meet with a macrobiotic teacher. I refused. I need to do this on my own — a teacher would only be another crutch — someone else to take responsibility for me. I needed to do this for me.

I continued to cook and eat, and things started to improve. Even my blood tests were beginning to reverse — ever so slightly. But that was enough to give me hope. I thought the worst was over. God, we can be so naive sometimes. To think that I could change my life so drastically with no payback was insane. But maybe it's better to be ignorant. The discharging began full force. First, the diarrhea which lasted a couple of weeks. I was so depleted, I thought I would never survive. Then my skin began to break out. The itching and erupting spread until I was completely covered with a rash. When that cleared (after eight weeks), I was left with a face full of pimples that would plague me for almost two years. Menstrual problems including an ovarian cyst developed. Hip baths and bancha tea douches solved that problem, only to be replaced by more discharging.

And so it went. Although the discharge was always unpleasant and almost impossible to bear, I knew I was improving. Each blood test revealed an improvement in my white cell count. The doctors were amazed. They called it "spontaneous regression" and said it was very rare — and could reverse at any time. I now know differently. Thirteen months after my practice of macrobiotics began, my white cell count was declared within normal range, where it has remained for almost seven years now.

And what did the doctors have to say now? Well, they said that spontaneous regression never yielded results like these, so this miraculous improvement had to be the result of something else. I then told them about macrobiotics. They called it voodoo and said it had nothing to do with my recovery. When I persisted, they said that I was probably misdiagnosed in the first place. I was blind with rage. I knew what I had just been through. Misdiagnosed? I was appalled at their arrogance and lack of vision. I left and have never returned.

When I began my practice of macrobiotics, I was going to eat and get well. The philosophy was of little interest to me. But as my health improved, so did my clarity and judgement. Even now, it seems as though the fog continues to disperse each day, and I wonder how I could have been blind to the order of the universe for so much of my life.

It is hard for me to remember the person I was before macrobiotics. Bob and I married and have created a wonderful life together. My gratitude to him is boundless; he was my teacher and my support system through the darkest times. We are the publishers of a newsletter — *Macro News* — that reaches many people in the Philadelphia area and around the world and is committed to sharing what we know to be the natural order. I work as a macrobiotic cook in a natural foods store and have begun to conduct cooking classes in our home (yes, my cooking improved dramatically since the beginning). I feel strong and my health continues to improve. Life is a wonder to me now.

People seem amazed when I tell them that cancer was the best thing to ever happened to me. Yet, without that trial, I would never have met my wonderful husband to whom I owe my very life. I never would have learned what true responsibility for oneself can mean. And chances are, I would have never discovered this way of life that has the potential of changing our entire civilization into what it was meant to be.

Source: Christina Pirello, "Macrobiotics: Getting Started," *Macro News*, Philadelphia, Pennsylvania, January/February, 1990.

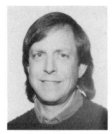

22.

Bill Templeton
Malignant Melanoma

In November 1986, at the age of thirty-two, my life in Huntsville, Texas, came to a sudden halt. I was diagnosed with Stage IV melanoma cancer on my lower right back. I went through the usual medical treatment of surgical removal followed by regular checkups. I was told not to worry. It's easy for someone else to say don't worry. Well, I began planning the end of my life, knowing Stage IV cancer is almost always fatal. I became a person living in fear.

Before I could finalize my plans, my marriage came to an end. I would lose the much needed support of my wife of ten years and my two-year-old daughter. I was forced to leave my family and business. I soon became involved in a Dallas business. So I moved to Dallas. I thought a new business would get the cancer and family problems off my mind. Perhaps even a miracle would take place driving the cancer out of my body.

Six months later my doctor found lumps in my groin area. He told me surgery was needed to find out what the lumps were. I went ahead with the surgery. The next day after surgery, I found out that the cancer had spread into my lymph system The doctor removed all the major lymph nodes in the area. He told me I needed eighty treatments of chemotherapy. I would have to stay in the hospital five days for each five treatments every two months. Each treatment lasted all day. I was told also I might need more surgery from time to time, followed by radiation treatments. Basically, I was not given much hope, only a 20 percent chance of survival with the treatments and no hope without them. I would also go through a lot of expense for these services. I began to think that I was surely a goner. I knew inside myself that there had to be a better way.

Then, all of a sudden, two days after surgery, my life changed again. It all started when an old college friend came to the hospital to visit me. He brought me a magazine article on the story of a man who recovered from cancer through the use of macrobiotics. The man's name was Dirk Benedict. Something instantly changed inside of me. I would never be the same person again. I knew I had found new hope for life, something I was drastically in need of.

I had never heard of macrobiotics. Growing up in Texas and living in a small town, you don't hear of such things. When you get sick you go to the doctor. You put your life in his hands. You don't understand you have to guide your own self back to health and happiness. I knew that macrobiotics would be my tool for recovery.

The next day I asked a member of my medical staff if he had heard of macrobiotics. He paused for a moment and went to close the door to my room. He then said, "Yes I have. But please promise me you will not mention our conversation to anyone." I said O.K. He began to tell me that he thought macrobiotics would work for some people. He said a person would have to be of the right character. Because of my willingness to think independently and my determination to live, he thought macrobiotics would work for me. He then gave me the names of two books he thought would help me. The books were *Recalled By Life* by Anthony Sattilaro, M.D., and *Confessions of a Kamikaze Cowboy* by Dirk Benedict. After three weeks in the hospital, I went to my mother's until I could go back to Dallas. After reading the books and returning to Dallas, I had my work cut out for me. I could barely get around, much less do all the things I would have to begin doing to get well.

Because of my serious condition, I had to jump right in to the macrobiotic diet. I would get up in the morning by 4:30, so I could fix my breakfast and do my stretching exercises, then go to work for about ten hours a day. I would force myself to walk after work for at least two miles. I would then go home and cook and chew my food at least 100 times a mouthful. I wanted to do everything right. I would go to bed usually around 11:00 P.M. which would give me three hours after eating before bedtime. On top of all this I would have to spend four hours a day for special treatments I needed, to help me get over the surgery. This took about five months.

After a few weeks on the macrobiotic diet, I started feeling the positive effects. My energy started going up and up. I soon started running and bicycling. Three months after surgery I managed to run over ten miles on some days. I wanted to beat the cancer and would do whatever it took to do so. Although I did take ten chemotherapy treatments, which was one of the worst experiences I have ever gone through, I soon totally walked away from all doctors and modern medicine. I decided I would take care of myself. I would take responsibility for my own life. For the first four months I learned everything about macrobiotics from books I would read. I developed the attitude that if macrobiotics did not work for me it would not work for anyone. I became very strong from my cooking and my new way of life. I would cut no corners.

After about five months of my new life I decided to go to Becket, Massachusetts, to attend a Macrobiotic Residential Seminar sponsored by the Kushi Institute. This was one of the greatest weeks of my life. It was like one big family there. I learned more in one week than I had in the past five months. I also met with a macrobiotic teacher and this helped me make more adjustments in my road to recovery. Following my visit, I decided to leave Dallas and move to Becket to work and live. A year later there were no signs of the cancer. Now, four years after being diagnosed with Stage IV melanoma, and receiving a negative prognosis for recovery, I feel stronger and better than I ever have in my life.

Source: Correspondence with Bill Templeton, Stockbridge, Massachusetts, November, 1990.

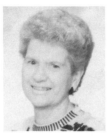

23.

Jean Bailey
Cancer of the Bile Duct and Pancreas

My fight with cancer began in 1963, when bleeding from one of my nipples sent me to a hospital in Windsor, Ontario. I was a busy mom with a seven-month-old baby girl, plus a five-year-old daughter and a four-year-old son.

A section of breast was surgically removed and the beginning of cancer cells were discovered. A simple mastectomy was immediately performed. My recovery was good and no chemotherapy was required. I was elated — I had won over cancer!

Life was good to me. I returned to caring for my family and the church work I enjoyed. Two more children were born to us, and I decided to return to work as a registered nurse in a nursing home.

Up to this point we had lived in a rented house at a seed corn plant where my husband, Doug, worked. Plant expansion, in 1975, forced us to plunge into debt and purchase our own home. Doug had been brought up to never buy anything that could not be paid for in cash outright. This was a tremendous step for him and one that was marked with increased stress on the both of us along with our family.

I was at that time working full time on the midnight shift which also contributed to the situation. I had been told that the only condition allowing a Christian wife and mother to work was that her family did not suffer. I was determined that mine would not. I tried to do everything as before — sewing, cleaning, redecorating, entertaining, keeping doctor appointments, and scheduled lessons for the children.

Life went on fairly well, I thought. However, a few years into this fast-paced lifestyle found me with increased blood pressure and medication for a heart problem, tension headaches and countless bottles of medication.

Doug accepted a job with another seed company in 1982, located approximately sixty miles away. We were moving again, but this time we were leaving close friends and all that was familiar to me. I had to give up my nighttime job which was a blessing in disguise, for soon my blood pressure returned to normal and I was off all medication.

I believed I was a good cook and provided my family with all the right foods. The children got their milk and lots of good protein (which, I believed, could only be found in red meats). We had our vegetables with lots of butter and, of course, dessert (my favorite).

When Doug's triglyceride level was discovered to be excessively elevated, he was told to cut down on red meats. I did not know how I would ever be able to cook a meal without hamburger, pork chops, or roasts, so I really did not cut back to any great extent.

We continued with this, our comfortable lifestyle, fully believing it was yielding good health. I first began to notice that I did not feel well in early autumn of 1987. I was irritable and tired and, as Christmas approached, I was constantly nauseated. The nausea increased if I ate rich or fried foods so I thought I had a problem with my gallbladder.

My doctor ordered tests which proved negative and since the family was returning home for Christmas, I did not think I had time to do anything about it. I had knitting to finish and all the traditional baking to get done. I enjoyed our Christmas together but often could not eat the meals I had prepared.

In January of 1988, I was back in the doctor's office. My urine had turned dark and I was sure I had something wrong with my liver. Blood work was done and I was soon hospitalized for more x-rays. Shortly thereafter, I was sent to a London, Ontario, hospital where many extensive, exhausting tests were performed, culminating with a MIR scan which pinpointed a tumor growing around the common bile duct.

The surgeon operated on January 15, hoping to be able to replace the bile duct with an internal tube but found that the cancer had destroyed the duct, plus taken hold in the pancreas and lymph glands. Thus, an external tube was put in place and I was returned to my room. Doug was informed of the details and told that I had about eight months to live — two months of fairly normal health and then rapid deterioration. One of the nurses told me to go home and enjoy my family.

Our eldest daughter, Darla, brought me Michio Kushi's book, *The Cancer-Prevention Diet*, and told me of a lady in her church who had a large cancerous growth on her scalp. She tried the macrobiotic diet and the cancer shrunk enough for it to be removed by doctors. Darla asked if I would be interested in trying it and I decided I had nothing to lose and everything to gain.

Darla called the Kushi Institute in Brookline, Massachusetts, which provided her Diane Silver Hassell's phone number. Diane lived near me and I visited with her on February 19 and began my macrobiotic journey.

Talk about a change! Everything I had known was put aside and my life was to start anew. I would have to learn to cook with grains, beans, and of all things — sea vegetables! We went shopping for things I could not even pronounce, let alone cook! Fears and feelings of inadequacies rushed in and I wondered if I could do all this.

I had tremendous support from my husband and family. Darla came home and emptied my cupboards of the things I would no longer use, replacing them with the grains and other foods we had bought. Doug bought me a new gas stove, as recommended, to replace the electric one. With this tremendous start, I was well on my way!

Tears of frustration ended many of my first cooking attempts. But with Doug encouraging me and with cooking lessons to help me, I finally started to enjoy the food and I could feel an improvement in my health. It is wonderful that a diet can do so much. I was told by my surgeon that I would experience severe back pain as the disease progressed but I have suffered no pain. My energy level has improved and I was soon back to work on a part time basis. Doug's triglyceride and cholesterol levels dropped low into the normal range. My doctor often asked what I was doing to look so good!

I am truly thankful for several things:

1. That I have a Heavenly Father who watches over me, keeps me and guides me.

2. For a loving husband and wonderful family who continue to pray for me.

3. For friends and a great church family who continue to pray for me.

4. For Diane and Dr. Chris Hassell who have taught and advised me, and for the macrobiotic diet that has helped to give me health and so far three very good years to enjoy, seeing two more of our children married and three more beautiful grandchildren.

The only regret I have, sad to say, is that more people who know of my illness and have seen my success of recovery do not wish to try it themselves.

Source: Correspondence with Jean Bailey, Ridgetown, Ontario, February, 1991.

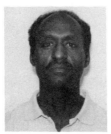

24.

Osbon Woodford
Colon Cancer

I am forty-four years old and I was born in Macon, Georgia, on November 8, 1946. The first twenty years of my life, I recall that nearly all the food I ate was homemade. However, this food was made with lard (hog fat), cooked in lard, and seasoned with grease left over from bacon or fat-back. Sugar in one form or another was also plentiful. Nevertheless, I maintained an average body weight of 170 pounds at 6' 1".

I spent my next twenty years eating food from all kinds of fast food locations and quick processed foods from supermarkets. Living on this kind of diet, I reached 210 pounds before my twenty-second birthday.

On April 10, 1987, I was diagnosed as having colon cancer. Two days later, I entered Riverside Methodist in Columbus, Ohio, and on April 16, I underwent surgery. The surgical pathology report stated the following: "Segment at sigmoid colon: poorly differentiated papillary adenocarcinoma with diffuse infiltration of the mesocolic fat, and metastasis to eleven lymph nodes including the highest lymph node at the vascular stalk."

The prognosis was gloomy. Eleven lymph nodes removed during surgery proved to be cancerous. I was a very high-risk patient, according to my oncologist; moreover, my wife was told that there was nothing that could be done for me. No chemotherapy, radiation, etc., was available, and the only thing recommended was that I brace myself for a recurrence somewhere in the brain, the lungs, or the liver within six months to a year.

On December 23, 1988, my oncologist advised me to have exploratory surgery because one of my crucial tests (Carcinoembryonic Antigen or CEA) had reached an alarming level. I made arrangements to undergo surgery at Ohio State University Hospital because surgeons there were using an experimental method of detecting cancerous tissues before they become so diseased as to be detected by the naked eye during exploratory surgery. While preparing for surgery, the test level declined back to normal levels and surgery was called off.

On February 27, 1990, after many normal low-level readings of the same CEA test, it became evident that I was stable and well, and my oncologist pronounced me "cured." According to him, my fast-growing cancer would have manifested itself already if it was going to reappear. Three years of uneventful good health had convinced him. He simply recommended that I continue doing whatever I was doing. A year later, on February 11, 1991, the same oncologist said that according to the medical statistics, I should not be alive. But I was in good health without a trace of cancer. And he repeated again that I should continue doing what I was doing.

What I had been doing for the past three years, and now four, was living the macrobiotic way. I never varied from a diet based around whole grains, vegetables, legumes, and sea vegetables. Along with my diet, I reduced my stress level markedly through reflection, meditation, and generally striving for more positive relationships and situations. Today I have a body weight of 150 lbs., a total cholesterol at 142 ("good" HDL cholesterol = 80; "bad" VLDL and LDL cholesterol = 62), and my blood is functioning at a level of 98 percent in terms of delivering oxygen to my body cells. I feel strong, happy, healthy, and I finally know what I felt for many months. I am free of cancer!

Source: Correspondence with Osbon Woodford, Columbus, Ohio, March, 1991.

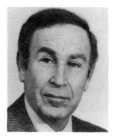

25.

Norman Arnold
Pancreatic Cancer

Nine years ago, Norman Arnold was diagnosed as having one of the most intractable of all malignancies: cancer of the pancreas with metastasis to the liver. At the age of fifty-two, Arnold was told by his physicians that he had perhaps four to nine months to live. Studies had shown that the mean life expectancy for those with pancreatic cancer is five months.

Today, Norman Arnold is well. According to numerous computed tomography (CT) scans, blood, ultrasound, and liver tests, he is completely free of cancer. His physicians are at a loss to explain his recovery. Indeed, Arnold abandoned conventional cancer therapies for alternative methods, including a macrobiotic diet.

On July 28, 1982, Norman Arnold entered the operating room at Providence Hospital in Columbia, South Carolina, expecting to undergo routine gallbladder surgery. During the operation, his surgeon, Dr. Dan Davis, discovered a large tumor on the head of his pancreas. He also found a smaller tumor in one of the lymph nodes and three cancerous lesions on Norman's liver. Apparently, the primary site of the cancer was the lymph nodes, with metastasis to the other locations. The tumor was biopsied and sent to pathology where it was diagnosed as adenocarcinoma, a highly virulent form of cancer. Davis realized that Norman was beyond remedial surgery. He removed his gallbladder and closed Arnold's abdomen.

Following the surgery, Norman and his wife, Gerry Sue, were told flatly that there was no cure for Norman's disease, nor was there any hope of recovery. Pancreatic cancer is one of the most devastating of all malignancies; it is thoroughly intractable to standard chemotherapy protocols and patients do not live long following diagnosis.

A lifelong resident of Columbia, South Carolina, Arnold is one of the state's leading businessmen and philanthropists; he has served on numerous local and statewide boards in medical care, job training programs, and other community service councils. In short, he was not accustomed to taking bad news passively.

He investigated all the medical and alternative cancer therapies, including interferon, hyperthermia treatment, radiation therapy, and a variety of experimental drugs. He subscribed to medical journals, newsletters, and computer information services. He searched the medical literature for every possible alternative to death. He also had the help of several physician-friends who assisted him in gathering research.

Of this varied and uncertain list of alternatives, two emerged to provide some hope. The first was macrobiotics, a diet and philosophy based on ancient principles developed in China some 2,500 years ago. The second was an experimental cancer treatment called monoclonal antibodies.

Norman was introduced to macrobiotics while still in the hospital recovering from the exploratory surgery that discovered his cancer. As he lay in his bed, still reeling from the devastating news, someone gave him a copy of the August 1982 issue of *Life Magazine.* In it was an excerpt from a forthcoming book entitled *Recalled By Life,* the story of a medical doctor's use of a macrobiotic diet to successfully treat his own cancer.

The macrobiotic diet is composed chiefly of whole grains, land

and sea vegetables, beans, fish, and fruit. The diet is low in fat and cholesterol and rich in all essential nutrients, including fiber. The philosophy includes the age-old concept of yin and yang, the ancient view that two opposite forces combine to create all phenomena. It is through balancing these two primordial forces that health is achieved.

Norman investigated macrobiotics and discovered that there were numerous accounts of people using the diet and lifestyle to overcome cancer. He was dubious, but intrigued. Arnold decided to have a friend, attorney John Rainey, investigate the claims. Rainey went through the files of the Kushi Institute and East West Foundation — both macrobiotic educational institutions located in Boston. He also searched the records of an Illinois medical doctor who used macrobiotics in his practice to help numerous people recover from serious illnesses, including cancer. Rainey then personally visited each person on record as having successfully dealt with cancer through the use of macrobiotics. Remarkably, the lawyer discovered that the vast majority of the claims were true; these people had in fact been diagnosed with terminal cancer and had used macrobiotics as their principal means of treatment.

Meanwhile, Norman's cousin, Dr. Charles Banov, an allergist and immunologist, was searching for medical treatments that might be of help to Norman. Banov soon discovered a highly experimental approach called monoclonal antibodies.

Monoclonal antibodies are proteins produced by the immune systems of mice to fight the type of cancer being dealt with by a human patient. The method works by injecting blood from the human patient into a mouse; the mouse creates an immune response, which doctors hope will be effective against the particular kind of cancer effecting the human patient. Once the immune system of the mouse has responded against the cancer, scientists extract the mouse antibodies and inject them into the patient in an attempt to stimulate the patient's immune system to produce an effective antibody against the malignancy.

In 1982, monoclonal antibodies had not been shown to be effective against any type of malignancy. (Monoclonal antibodies remain an unproven therapy against cancer to this day. No study has proven that they are effective in the treatment of cancer.)

Norman decided to use both the macrobiotic diet and the antibodies.

In August 1982, Gerry Sue, their three sons, and Norman began the macrobiotic diet.

A month later, Norman was given an injection of the monoclonal antibodies, which were produced by scientists at Wistar Institute in Philadelphia, Pennsylvania, a branch of the University of Pennsylvania Medical School. There would be only one injection. He would simply have to wait to see what effect the antibodies had, if any.

Arnold would not stop there. He intended to employ any treatment that offered the least bit of hope, with the minimum of side effects.

At the Vince Lombardi Cancer Center at Georgetown, Dr. Phillip Schein was studying a combination of chemotherapy drugs against pancreatic cancer. Schein is regarded as one of the two leading figures in pancreatic research in the United States and among a handful of leading specialists in the world. That September, Norman began taking the chemotherapy protocol under Schein's direction.

Arnold underwent five treatments of chemotherapy. The effects of the drugs were devastating: weight loss, chronic fatigue, muscle wasting, nausea, and total loss of body hair. His weight dropped from 160 to 112 pounds. He looked like a refugee from Auschwitz. At times, he became despondent. By the time fall arrived, he wondered what good the chemotherapy might be doing for him, and why he was even subjecting himself to such treatment.

Norman, Gerry Sue, and their three boys went to the Bahamas for Thanksgiving, 1982. There, amidst the natural beauty of the island and his family's love, Norman continued to question the use of chemotherapy for his disease. Dr. Schein had made it clear that the chemotherapy was not a cure; it wasn't even a guarantee of a few more months. Nevertheless, Schein wanted Norman to take the chemotherapy as long as he was able. The doctor had hoped that by continually bombarding the cancer, the drugs might slow the growth of the tumor and extend Norman's life. But what sort of life did the chemotherapy offer? Norman was wasting away. One of the most painful experiences for Norman was seeing the pity in the faces of his friends. It wasn't just sadness people were communicating; virtually everyone he knew believed he was far beyond hope.

"I'd rather die in some more dignified way than have my sons remember me like this," Arnold said.

At the same time, the macrobiotic approach had begun to appeal to him. Norman had long been fascinated by nutrition, though his previous interest focused exclusively on vitamin therapy. But the macrobiotic idea that diet and lifestyle were the leading factors in both the onset and recovery of disease struck a deep chord in him. On that Thanksgiving holiday, Norman decided to quit the chemotherapy and commit himself exclusively to the macrobiotic regimen.

Meanwhile, he continued searching for answers.

In November, Gerry Sue and Norman attended a five-day seminar at the Simonton Clinic in Dallas, Texas, famous for its successful use of mental imagery in the treatment of cancer. Under the direction of Stephanie Simonton, wife of the clinic's founder, Dr. O. Carl Simonton, Norman and Gerry Sue learned of the importance of the mind in the maintenance and enhancement of the immune system.

Mental imagery became a fundamental part of Norman's daily health routine. Among the images he used was the picture of his tumor being eroded by his blood, now strengthened thanks to his macrobiotic regimen.

Norman was guided through the uncertainty and conflicting data by two men, one a medical doctor, the other a philosopher and teacher of macrobiotics. The medical doctor was Charles Banov, Norman's cousin and boyhood friend. The macrobiotic teacher was Michio Kushi, a man of rare insight and wisdom who used the methods of Eastern philosophy and medicine to help restore Norman's health. These two men represented the best of West and East, modern and traditional medicine.

Kushi's ideas were particularly challenging. The macrobiotic philosophy maintained that the typical American diet, rich in fat, cholesterol, sugar, refined grains, and chemicals, provided an onslaught of poisons that, once inside the body, accumulated into masses. These accumulated toxins prevented adequate blood flow to organs and tissues, suffocating and deforming cells. A variety of ill-nesses began to manifest as a result, including heart disease, dia-betes, and arthritis. By depriving tissues of oxygen and, at the same time, polluting the cellular environment with toxins, the daily diet also affected the DNA, or genetic material, of cells. Once the DNA was altered, cells often began to multiply out of control, thus be-coming cancerous.

Kushi maintained, however, that by eating a diet that is free of these toxins, and at the same time rich in nutrients, the body can throw off the accumulated poisons and restore balance and health. This "throwing off" of waste was typically referred to in macrobio-tics as "discharging."

Once he began the diet, Norman indeed began to discharge. He lost weight and suffered a variety of passing cold symptoms. One of the most frightening of all was that his tongue turned black. He awoke one morning, opened his mouth to brush his teeth, and no-ticed that his tongue had turned black. Gerry Sue was aghast. She called Michio in a panic. Kushi calmly reassured her that Norman's tongue would regain its normal color, and that it was a good sign. Norman's system was deeply cleansing itself. In fact, the tongue's normal color did return, but the experience was terrifying.

Gerry Sue was regularly calling Michio to say that Norman was steadily losing weight. Kushi reassured her each time that even-tually Norman's weight would stabilize and he would even regain a few pounds once he reached optimal weight. This, too, came to pass.

Following his diagnosis of cancer, Norman had a CT scan per-formed that clearly detected the cancerous tumors on his pancreas and liver. But in the months that followed, Norman felt stronger, more vital, and more alive than he had felt in many years. There was no doubt in his mind that the diet was having a profound effect on every aspect of his life: mental clarity improved; energy greatly increased; his weight stabilized and reached an optimum level.

On June 24, 1983, just nine months after he was diagnosed and began the macrobiotic diet, Norman had another CT scan per-formed, this one showing only the faint presence of the tumors. They had clearly begun to shrink.

On December 21, 1983, another CT scan was unequivocal: All clear! The test revealed no presence of cancer. Numerous other examinations followed, including blood, ultrasound, and liver tests, all of which showed no sign of cancer anywhere in Norman's body. His doctors were baffled. Norman was triumphant.

On his sixtieth birthday in January 1990, Norman climbed Mount Kilimanjaro, whose peak stands at 19,600 feet above sea level. He continues to be an avid tennis player and scuba diver.

In the spring of 1991 — the time of this writing — Norman Arnold remained in excellent health. His doctors remain at a loss to explain his recovery.

Source: *The Norman Arnold Story: Conquering Cancer of the Pancreas*, by Tom Monte.

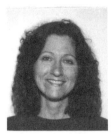

26.

Emily Bellew
Hodgkin's Disease

I was twenty-two years old and I had been married for three years. We were expecting our first child, a baby that was going to add so much to our beginning. We had so much hope for the future. Little did I know all this was going to be very short-lived.

I had a very difficult preganancy and delivery, and on top of all of this I had gained eighty pounds. I weighed 205 the day I delivered. From the moment that I was nine days pregnant I craved food, all kinds of food. My appetite was never satisfied. From morning till night I ate. I was eating sweets and ice cream in large amounts, along with red meat and anything else I could get my hands on. I didn't feel well after Bryan was born, but to me this was no surprise. The surprise was that as soon as I delivered it seemed that my uncontrollable appetite diminished.

Three days after Bryan was born I was annoyed by a swollen and stiff neck. I attributed this to holding Bryan in the wrong position as I walked him nights to get him to sleep. After his sleeplessness subsided, the condition with my neck did not. Three weeks later I decided to go for my postpartum checkup a few weeks early because I just did not feel well and was always tired. The doctor examined me and said all seemed O.K. I was ready to go home when my husband mentioned to him the stiffness and swelling in my neck. The doctor took one look and phoned another doctor at Ohio University which was an hour drive from our home. My doctor gave me his name and sent us home with an appointment set up in Columbus three days later. I thought this was all pretty silly just for a stiff neck and I really thought he was crazy when I looked in a dictionary and discovered that an oncologist was a doctor that dealt with cancer.

Three days later we were on our way to Columbus. I was prepared for the doctor wanting to keep me overnight, but never anticipated that I would be there slightly over one month. As soon as I registered and got my room a whirlwind of tests began. Tests in, on and around my body, these people were looking at things in my body I didn't even know I had, let alone knowing there was some type of strange, sometimes painful test for it.

This went on for three days. On the third day a surgeon came to see me; he wanted to operate and see what was causing my neck to swell. Less than an hour later I was in the operating room. I chose to do the operation under a local anesthetic; I was assured this was very routine and would only take 15 or 20 minutes. One and a half hours later they began to stitch me up. I heard the doctor ask for a frozen section; the only thing that came to my mind was a dairy queen. They finally finished and I was taken to my room. A few hours later the surgeon returned and told me it would take three days to confirm, but he was sure I had a type of cancer called Hodgkin's Disease. I was numb; all I wanted was for this to be over and get home to my son.

The three-day wait ended and it was confirmed that I did have Hodgkin's Disease. Hodgkin's Disease is a cancer that strikes many young adults between the ages of eighteen and twenty-five. Hodgkin's has four stages ranging from one to four. It is believed that the early stage (Stage I) starts in the lymph glands above the shoulders, Stage II is when it spreads below the neck but above the diaphragm, Stage III is below the diaphragm, and Stage IV, being the worst, is in the bone. I was Stage II-B, B meaning I had symptoms (A is when the patient shows no symptoms). These symptoms can be such things as: itching skin, weight loss, fatigue — just to mention a few.

For the next month I put myself into the hands of the doctors and went along for the ride. After many more tests and another operation to see if the cancer had spread below the neck, the decision was made to try to eradicate the cancer with radiation treatments. I came home and began my treatments that lasted six months. I remember the last day — it was a dreary, rainy summer afternoon and I thought it the most beautiful day I had ever seen.

The next few months were wonderful, but this didn't last for long; the worst thing that could happen did. The cancer returned and this time it showed up in the ischium, which is the lower portion of the hip bone, eating away about one quarter inch of it. That is how I ended up in a wheelchair for about five months unable to walk. I also started chemotherapy. Seven months later I ended treatments and the bone had healed. I couldn't wait to get on with my life which had been on hold now for almost fifteen months. My son was growing and he was a joy to be around. He made me laugh every day. My whole family was supportive and was there by my side.

I wish this was the end of my story and I could say we lived happily ever after, but again I was free of the cancer for only a few months. A tumor started to grow in my abdomen; again I began chemo. Another seven months passed and again it was over. Please let this time be the last. They told me if I get it again there would be no treatments left for me. I grew up so much from the girl that entered the hospital almost two and a half years before. I became more independent, confident, and even happier than I ever was before. I didn't let my illness get me down, and I discovered how strong and resilient I was. I started to take charge of my life and pay a lot more attention to my health.

Six months passed. I was enjoying each hour not wanting to waste a moment. I wanted to take in all life had to offer. I wasn't feeling for any lumps when I took my shower that morning, but it was there. I couldn't deny it. A small lump in the groin area this time. What was I going to do? I received all the treatments they use to fight my disease and my doctor confirmed this. I wouldn't give up. I would keep on looking and looking I did. First, I tried to get into St. Judes, but I was too old. Then I treid the National Cancer Institute in Boston. Again, I was rejected because I had already had treatments. Next my husband and I started off for John Hopkins in Baltimore; there they told me that they could offer me chemo. That would cure me or kill; I wasn't ready for that yet. From there we went back home and flew to Stanford University in Palo Alto, California. That is where I found a doctor who set up a new type of chemo for me and arranged for Columbus University to administer it. Also this is where I bought a book called *Recalled By Life*.

Back to Columbus we came and started treatments. One month later I was back again for the second dose. It was my twenty sixth birthday, one that I will never forget. It started out with my Hickman catheter plugging up. They worked on it for what seemed to be hours. This is when my doctor said it wouldn't matter much if I received the treatment or not because it would do little good. It might stretch my life a few more months if any. He said I would be lucky to be alive in a year. With this I got up, packed my bags and went home.

A few days later I finished *Recalled By Life*. I had read dozens of other books on diet and cancer and never gave them much more thought. What I read about macrobiotics in this book made me want to learn more. I couldn't find any other information at the library or the book store. Next, I called the publisher who gave me the number to the Kushi Institute in Boston. I was told that a man named Michio Kushi was traveling around as we spoke, giving seminars. His next seminar was to begin in Cincinnati and last for three days. This was only three hours away, so I packed my bags and took off for Cincinnati. The next three days changed my life. I heard lectures and attended cooking classes. I also began to eat macrobiotic food for the first time. I took new knowledge and new cookbooks back home and began cooking. I started to feel the difference right away and it was all so really simple. This was the way our bodies were meant to be nourished. Weeks went by and then months and finally a year. I felt better than I ever had even before I became sick. The doctors had no answers except that it was a miracle that the tumor went away, giving no credit to macrobiotics. Two more years passed. I felt fine and healthy and was maintaining my weight at 113 pounds. It was now four years that I was eating this way and feeling so good I began to slip back into eating a few bad foods on a regular basis, like chicken and salad oils. Slowly over the next four years I added more and more unhealthy foods one by one until finally it began to catch up with me. I had little energy. I gained twenty pounds and I was looking and feeling very unhealthy. I never want to go through having cancer again, but I felt this was where I was heading. Once again I have turned back to macrobiotics. Just recently I returned from Becket, Massachusetts, at the Kushi Institute where I spent one week brushing up on my cooking skills, listening to lectures and enjoying macrobiotic cuisine. One month has passed and I am already beginning to feel better and taking off the weight I had gained. It will be awhile until I once again feel my best but as each day goes by I feel stronger and have more energy. I've eaten both ways and I know from here on I choose to eat macrobiotically for both my health and happiness. This August I will be thirty-four and in December Bryan will be thirteen. Nine years have passed since I walked away from the hospital.

Source: Correspondence with Emily Bellew, Zanesville, Ohio, April, 1991.

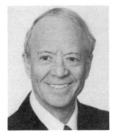

27.

Bill Garnell
Prostate Tumor

On July 14, 1988, during a routine company examination, the examining physician discovered a nodule on Bill Garnell's prostate. He suggested that Bill, an executive for American Telegraph and Telephone, visit a urologist to confirm his findings. On July 20, a physician in Morristown, N.J., confirmed the previous diagnosis and suggested he go for an immediate biopsy to determine whether it was malignant.

Bill declined. During the 1970s, he had become familiar with the macrobiotic way of life and with the possibility of recovering from serious illness through a change in diet and lifestyle He immediately set up a personal educational interview with educator Michio Kushi.

On August 11, 1988, after meeting with Mr. Kushi and Edward Esko, a senior macrobiotic teacher at the Kushi Institute in Boston, he began the standard macrobiotic diet with personal modifications, including three special drinks and additional practices such as scrub-ing his body and soaking his feet to stimulate energy flow. Along with his wife, Natalie, he began to study the theory of macrobiotics, and Natalie took macrobiotic cooking lessons with Suzanne Landry, a Kushi Institute graduate in Morristown. "We both knew in our hearts we were pursuing the right course in healing my cancer," Bill recalled.

On April 10, 1989, bowing to pressure from his family for a medical opinion, Bill underwent a complete urological examination by the head of the Urology Department in Newark, N.J. "He found absolutely no evidence of any nodule on my prostate," Bill reported.

"We were elated! All the many hours we have spent cooking, scrubbing, soaking, and praying have proved that the macrobiotic concept of healing is valid. We are most grateful to Michio and the macrobiotic community for their support during the past year. We joyfully continue to spread our good news to family and friends in the hope that others will choose the same road we have taken."

Source: "Executive Recovers from Prostate Cancer," *One Peaceful World* Newsletter, Autumn, 1989.

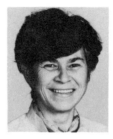

28.

Milenka Dobic
Ovarian and Lymph Cancer

In 1987, tragedy struck Milenka Dobic and her family. She was diagnosed with a metastasized uterine cancer and given two months to live by her doctors. Today Milenka seems to have unlimited resources of energy, she likes to sing while she cooks in the kitchen, she is vibrant with life, and because of her determination, the whole health of her country, Yugoslavia, may very well change.

Milenka and her husband, Bosko, are in their mid-forties. They have two children, a teenage son, Srdjan, and a daughter, Jelena, who is in grade school. Until 1986, they seemed to be, in all respects, a perfect example of a happy modern family. Both Mikenka and her husband were very successful in their professions. Milenka had a challenging and interesting career as the program director of one of the most important radio stations in Yugoslavia. Bosko was in the field of importing and exporting agricultural machinery.

In 1985, however, Milenka started having problems with her health: migraine headaches, constant tiredness, and pressure in her head. Since she had a very busy schedule and frenetic life, working long hours, Milenka first attributed these symptoms to "stress." After a few months, she decided to go to the hospital for a check-up. The doctors could not detect anything wrong and attributed her problems to aging! Nobody asked her questions about her diet. Milenka went back to work, but the pains seemed to increase until, one day, she felt so weak at work that she was unable to move. She went back to the hospital for more extensive tests and exams. A malignant tumor was discovered on her left ovary and, by that time, the cancer had already spread to the lymph system. From then on, things went very fast. Milenka was immediately operated on and underwent a total hysterectomy. A few days after the operation, however, her doctors told her that they had not been able to remove all of the tumor, and they advised chemotherapy and radiation.

At that point, Milenka decided it was time to take her destiny into her own hands. During her hospitalization, she had gathered information about her disease and the prognosis of similar cases. She never resigned herself to the role of passive victim. She first realized that the kind of tumor she had did not respond well to chemotherapy. As she was seeking information, Dr. Radka Rudic, a close friend of hers, recommended that she read *The Cancer-Prevention Diet* by Michio Kushi and *Recalled by Life* by Anthony Sattilaro, M.D., which had just been translated into Yugoslavian and linked cancer to faulty nutrition.

Milenka read the books and made up her mind. She was convinced that the cause of her cancer lay in her past history of eating meat, dairy, and oily foods, and that it could also be reversed by diet. She told her doctors that she would sign for her release and go back home. The doctors then warned her husband that if she left the hospital, she could not be expected to live more than two months. Milenka, however, had no intention to die: "My reaction all along was, I love this life, this world," she recalls. "It is impossible for me to leave now." At home, she gathered her family and told her children that she had cancer. "But I also said to them, 'We have to fight back.'" She announced her intention to go the the United States and learn more about macrobiotics. "We were really pioneers. There was no macrobiotic community or support in Yugoslavia at that time. But I had decided that macrobiotics would be my way of life as well as my family's. I was determined."

Milenka had always had many friends, and their friendship and sense of solidarity proved to be priceless in that difficult time. When her colleagues learned of her decision, they organized a radio program and fund-raising in her name. Thanks to her friends, colleagues, and listeners, who all supported her morally and financially, Milenka arrived in Boston in February, 1987, accompanied by her husband, Bosko, who had supported her decision all along.

"It was like a dream. We really didn't know where we were going or exactly what we were going to do. But there we were in Boston. When we arrived, though, we discovered that a two-day Way of Life Seminar was about to start with Michio Kushi and that we would be able to arrange a consultation with him. We were lucky."

During her visit with Michio Kushi, Milenka came to see that her cancer was caused by her past intake of food, especially cheese and dairy products, and that she could recover if she followed the macrobiotic dietary recommendations. "At that moment," she looks back, "I felt like my journey was really starting. I had hope now."

Bosko, aware that family support was essential for recovery, also changed his way of eating and started practicing macrobiotics himself. Milenka took several cooking classes and helped in the kitchen at the Kushi Institute. After thirteen days, they had to return home. But one problem remained: "There was no macrobiotic store to buy food in Yugoslavia. So we bought all kinds of cooking utensils and a six-months' supply of food." Needless to say, their luggage was very, very heavy!

Back home, Milenka started cooking for herself. Her husband and a friend of hers, a doctor, would start translating recipes from Aveline Kushi's cookbook at 6 A.M. and Milenka would practice her cooking. At the beginning, she had very little energy and could hardly stand or sit. Very quickly, though, her energy started increasing. With amazing will and self-discipline, Milenka then started a very strict schedule. She would get up at 5 A.M. and start her day with meditation, do-in massage, and body scrub, and start cooking at 9. "There was not a moment when I was not thinking of getting better, in all kinds of ways. I would sing songs. I would visualize my body, and there were two parts: a white half and a dark half. Every day, the bright part was becoming bigger. Wanting to be healthy was not just a sentence for me! It was a very deep feeling."

Every month, she would go to the hospital for blood tests and medical exams, and every month the results were better. After five months, the tumor had disappeared. "To the doctors, it seemed like a miracle. They could not understand."

Little by little, people heard of her case, and all the listeners who had participated in the fund raisings wanted to know what was going on. She was interviewed for different newspapers, magazines, radio, and TV stations. A special radio program was even broadcast from Milenka and Boskos' home with the participation of Dr. Miladin Mirilov, a vice-president of the World Health Organization, Sofia Borovnica, a member of the Parliament, and Dr. Drago Kovacevic, President of the Committee for Ecology in the government. Since her story had also appeared in newspapers distributed in foreign countries, people started calling the Dobics from all over the world. Milenka was able to arrange two other meetings with Michio Kushi, one in Switzerland and one in Yugoslavia in April, 1988, when Mr. Kushi was officially invited to Yugoslavia, following a growing interest in macrobiotics. At that meeting, Michio talked with Milenka, shook her hand, and said, "Congratulations, Milenka."

"I had won! I was so elated!"

Milenka immediately called her friends at the radio station, and another program was broadcast all over the country.

Michio Kushi's trip to Yugoslavia was also a great success. He met with some 300 doctors in Zagreb and 500 in Belgrade. In each city, forums were organized, each attended by over a thousand people. In each forum, he introduced the macrobiotic view and approach to disease and modern problems. He was also welcomed by the Committee of Agriculture of the Yugoslavian parliament and met with 200 agricultural leaders. At each public conference Milenka was invited to tell her story.

Meanwhile, the life of the whole family underwent tremendous changes. Milenka slowly introduced her two children to macrobiotics, taking out first meat, then dairy food from their diet, and replacing them with seitan, tempeh, and better quality foods. "My mother is very strong," says her son, Srdjan, who subsequently graduated from the Leadership Training Program of the Kushi Institute in Boston. "She managed to include us. She knew how to." Her husband also perceived changes, "We became much closer, more of a unit. I started to know intuitively when I should call home and check on my family."

Who says faith cannot move mountains?

Source: Adapted from Liliane Papin, Ph.D., "Life Is a Phoenix: A Yugoslavian Family's Triumph Over Cancer," *Return to Paradise*, Spring, 1989.

Part III
Medical Research

Summary of
A Retrospective Study of
Diet and Cancer
of the Pancreas

The following is a brief summary of "A Retrospective Study of Diet and Cancer of the Pancreas," a study of macrobiotics and cancer carried out at Tulane School of Public Health and Tropical Medicine (Department of Nutrition) in 1984/85.

Purpose

The purpose of this study was to determine whether pancreatic cancer patients who adopted macrobiotic diets survived longer than those who did not.

Methods

The study sampling frame consisted of all patients with primary cancer of the pancreas who received macrobiotic dietary counseling during the period January 1, 1980, through June 30, 1984, from a counselor listed in the *1984-85 Worldwide Macrobiotic Directory* (published by the East West Foundation, Brookline, Mass.).

Subjects include those individuals from this sampling frame who (or whose next-of-kin), when contacted, reported that they had followed a macrobiotic diet for at least three months.

Controls consisted of pancreatic cancer cases from the SEER (*S*urveillance *E*pidemiology and *E*nd *R*esults) national tumor registry diagnosed during the same time period.

Pathological confirmation of the disease and the date of diagnosis was obtained, when possible, from the subject's physician and/or the hospital medical records department. In cases where the medical records or pathology report could not be obtained, the patient or next-of-kin was asked to confirm the disease site and date of diagnosis. Date of death was requested from the next-of-kin.

Results

The sampling frame consisted of 110 individuals. Only thirty-seven out of the 110 patients (or next-of-kin) could be reached. Of these, twenty-four reported that they had practiced macrobiotics to a moderate or great extent for at least three months. Pathological confirmation could not be obtained for the majority of these cases. Nonetheless, survival analyses are based on these twenty-four macrobiotic pancreatic cancer patients.

The mean length of survival in the twenty-four patients was 17.3 months, compared with 6.0 months for the SEER patients. Median survival was 13.0 months vs. 3.0 months for SEER. The one-year survival rate was 54.2 percent (13/24) in the macrobiotic patients vs. 10.0 percent (950/9500) for SEER patients. All three comparisons were statistically significant (x2 tests resulted in p-values < .01).

Conclusions

While these findings are suggestive of an effect of macrobiotic practice on survival in pancreatic cancer, no firm conclusions can be drawn for several reasons:

1. There was a high non-response rate and incomplete medical confirmation of cases.

2. Ambulatory patients were disproportionately represented in the macrobotic group. Innate "hardiness," rather than dietary chang-

es, may have accounted for survival differences.

3. Attitudinal change (rather than dietary change) may have been the "active ingredient."

Further research is clearly warranted. Subject randomization, close dietary monitoring, rigorous disease documentation, and biological and quality of life endpoints should be employed in future studies.

Note: One of the researchers involved with this study is currently researching diet and breast cancer at the University of Michigan and working with Tulane investigators on two matched case-control studies of macrobiotics: one with pancreatic cancer and one with prostate cancer.

Remission of Advanced Malignant Disease: A Review of Cases with a Possible Dietary Factor by Vivien Newbold, M.D.

Dedication

This article is dedicated to Michio Kushi, the macrobiotic counselors and the entire macrobiotic community, in sincere appreciation for their courage and wisdom in bringing macrobiotics to so many whose lives have been transformed for the better.

Introduction

In December 1983, my husband was found to have terminal, medically incurable metastatic colon cancer, and was given only four to six months to live. As a physician I knew modern medicine could do nothing to save him. At best, it might slightly prolong his life at the cost of all the side effects of chemotherapy. Having grown up in the Orient, I had seen people who had used various Chinese approaches recover from illnesses that modern medicine has no idea how to cure. Thus we knew that if one form of healing didn't work, we could try another. We turned to macrobiotics.

Many of my colleagues thought I was crazy. "How can you feed him that stuff in his dying days?" they would ask, as they showed me article after article stating emphatically, ". . . after a careful search of the literature, there are no documented cases of recovery from cancer using the macrobiotic diet." Furthermore, many learned writers cited the extreme danger of malnutrition on the macrobiotic diet. But every day, instead of dying my husband was looking stronger and healthier. Macrobiotics seemed to be working. I vowed that if he recovered I would document his case and submit it to a medical journal for publication. I was sure they would want to know of his recovery.

In July 1984, eight months after his case was described as hopeless, not only was my husband feeling healthier than he had ever felt in his life, but a follow-up CT scan revealed that about 70 percent of the cancer was gone! I was beside myself with excitement. Some 60,000 people a year in the United States alone die from metastatic colon cancer, and the medical profession has openly stated it has made no significant progress in the treatment of colon cancer in more than fifty years. With this in mind, I called the American Cancer Society to let them know the wonderful news. I asked to speak to the director. I was shocked when I heard him say "It is of no interest to us." Well, I thought, maybe it was of no interest to him, but perhaps the NIH, and the National Cancer Institute would like to know. They too responded, "It is of no interest to us."

I could not believe that the medical institutions of our country really weren't interested; perhaps they just needed to hear of more than one case, and in writing. So, at great personal expense, I set about finding medically incurable cases that had recovered using macrobiotics. With the help of one of my colleagues, we carefully documented six such cases, and submitted them in an article to the *New England Journal of Medicine* for publication. We were sure the editors of this well known medical journal would want the rest of the world to know, however strange it was, a small group of people had experienced total regression of medically incurable cancer while using a dietary approach to creating good health. I was deeply shocked when I received their response, "It's of insufficient interest to our readership."

I refused to believe our medical institutions, filled with dedicated scientists, did not want to know there might be an inexpensive way to heal a disease that is killing one in five Americans every year. I decided perhaps my article documenting these cases might not have been written well enough. After all, I am an emergency room physician and not a professional scientist. Once again, this time with the assistance of a professional medical research writer, I rewrote the paper and submitted it to the *Lancet* and later to the *Journal of the American Medical Association.* Both, to my astonishment and dismay, replied it was of insufficient interest to their readership.

What does all this mean? Does the medical profession really want to know if there is a possible way to cure cancer, or do they just want to keep funding a system that clearly has made next to no progress in the treatment of most cancers in the last fifty years? They state repeatedly in their articles that a careful review of their literature reveals there are no documented cases of recovery using macrobiotics, and further, macrobiotics is nutritionally unsound and potentially dangerous. Of what use is a careful review of their literature if medical journals refuse to publish any cases indicating macrobiotics, or any other unconventional approach to healing for that matter, may have played an important role? Are our major scientific institutions made up of scientists who truly want to heal cancer? Isn't it strange these great institutions had no interst in reviewing the cases, going over the pathology slides, the x-rays and so on? Isn't it strange they had no interest in examining these patients carefully to look for the development of special antibodies that could help better understand regression of cancer? What kind of scientists do we have working in these major institutions?

If you were to stand on the street corner of any major city in the world and ask "Do you know of anyone who has recovered from a medically incurable disease using an unconventional approach?" how many cases do you think you would have by the end of one day? Do you think you would hear of a number of remedies that might be of some benefit to society? How many cases have to be presented, and in what form do they have to appear before the medical establishment will begin to consider other possibilities exist?

For the last few years my paper has sat gathering dust until I finally realized I was trying to share this valuable information with the wrong group of people. I realized this information needs to be shared with the people who want it. Therefore, I have rewritten much of the article, adding as much information as possible to make it as helpful as I know how to the average person. However, I have left the actual documentation of the cases in their original form, so anyone with a knowledge of medicine can benefit from reading the actual cases. I hope this article will assist you. And I hope that if you or someone you love is facing a challenging illness, it will lead you to a path of healing with joy.

Article

In this article, I present six case histories of patients with advanced, medically incurable cancer who used the macrobiotic approach to creating health and experienced complete regression of their cancers. In each case the regression could not have been due to any conventional medical treatment the patient received. These cases and others like them certainly do not prove that macrobiotics cured the patients; however, they clearly raise important questions which the medical profession might seriously consider. For example, can macrobiotics be of benefit to patients with cancer when medical treatment cannot help?

The macrobiotic approach to creating health encompasses every aspect of a person's life. It is based on the Oriental philosophy that each of us is reponsible for creating everything in our lives, including our illnesses. This is not from a standpoint of guilt, but rather of power. If we created it, then we have the power to change it.

Traditional Oriental philosophy views all of nature as consisting of two fundamental and opposing forces. Within each of us, the more balanced the state of these opposing forces, the higher the person's state of health and well being. The goal of macrobiotics is to bring every aspect of life — including exercise, work, environment, and especially diet —into harmony and balance.

A cornerstone of macrobiotics states: our thoughts and beliefs create our reality. We choose the foods we eat, how we prepare them, eat them and digest them in a manner which unconciously supports these thoughts and beliefs. If we dwell on recurrent negative thoughts such as resentment, then the food we eat transforms these thoughts into form which over time can present itself as disease. The exact disease we create depends on a wide combination of factors, the most important of which are our beliefs, recurrent thought patterns, underlying constitution, and the foods we eat. Macrobiotics views the patient as the master of his or her own destiny. When patients gain an understanding of the underlying causes of the imbalances they have created, then they have the opportunity to change and restore harmony and balance into their lives.

Central to macrobiotics is the understanding of the powerful effects of different foods on the body. Since each of us is unique, the ideal diet for each person is different and varies according to each person's way of life, goals, constitution, weather conditions, season of the year, present location, etc. However, so that the reader has some reference point, it is reasonable to say in general, the average macrobiotic person's diet consists of 50 to 60 percent whole cereal grains, 5 percent soups, 25 to 30 percent vegetables, and 5 to 10 percent beans and sea vegetables, plus occasional seafood, seasonal fruits, nuts and seeds. Chemically treated or highly processed foods are generally avoided, as is cooking with electricity.

This bare outline in no way reflects the immense diversity that is found in macrobiotic diets. There is no such thing as a single, all-purpose macrobiotic diet. Heavy physical exercisers have completely different needs, for example, than those sitting quietly all day. Similarly, those with terminal illnesses have very special requirements and need enormous variety in their meals. For those interested in gaining a more in depth understanding of macrobiotic cooking, there are many excellent macrobiotic cookbooks available, such as Aveline Kushi and Wendy Esko's book *Macrobiotic Family Favorites* and *A Complete Guide to Macrobiotic Cooking* by Aveline Kushi. The best way to get an understanding of macrobiotic cooking is to attend cooking classes given by a certified macrobiotic cooking instructor in your area.

Patients with serious illnesses need to see a macrobiotic counselor, who will evaluate the patient's condition on the basis of traditional Oriental methods of diagnosis. The patient is usually given a very precise diet — unique to that person — which frequently excludes many foods found in typical macrobiotic diets, and adds a number of specially prepared foods. The patient requires food cooked with care and with as thorough an understanding of macrobiotics as possible. Typically, the macrobiotic counselor evaluates the patient every four to six weeks and adjustments are made to the diet. Macrobiotics does not include the use of vitamin supplements, and none of the patients in this article took any. All the patients (except E and F) reported here adhered to their prescribed diets without any deviation. Because each patient's diet was especially formulated, the individual diet plans have not been included in the case histories.

How the Cases Were Found

With the invaluable assistance of a friend, David Westwater, all the macrobiotic centers within the United States were asked for the names and addresses of any cases of patients with medically incurable illnesses who had recovered or done extraordinarily well using macrobiotics. If the case was promising, the patient was contacted and asked if they would be part of the study. The patient signed a release for their hospital records and agreed to have their case published. There were several patients with advanced cancer who had completely recovered using macrobiotics who refused to release their records.

Although there were a quite a number of patients with a wide variety of illnesses who had done extraordinarily well, only those patients with no other possible explanation for their recovery were reported in this study. All cases of patients with prostate cancer were referred to Professor James Carter of Tulane University for evaluation in a separate study. Finally, very narrow criteria for inclusion in this article were used so as to present only the most impressive cases. These criteria were (1) the patient must have had biopsy-proven, advanced, medically incurable cancer, and the biopsy had to be available for inspection (there were two dramatic cases in which we had the biopsy report, but the hospital lost the actual biopsy); (2) after using the macrobiotic approach, the patient must have had no detectable sign of cancer. There were many cases in which the cancer decreased in size, or the patient had greatly outlived the prognosis, but they were not included. And (3) the regression of the cancer could not have been attributable to any conventional medical therapy the patient received.

Case Histories

Case A

Patient A is a sixty-one year old white male who complained of increasingly severe epigastric discomfort and underwent surgery at Providence Hospital, Columbia, South Carolina, on July 28, 1982, for suspected chronic cholecystitis and cholelithiasis. At surgery, he was found to have an adenocarcinoma of the head of the pancreas with metastasis to the iliac node and an isolated 1.2 cm metastasis to the liver. Biopsy specimens of the lymph node and liver lesion were taken and both confirmed the diagnosis of metastatic adenocarcinoma of the pancreas.

Preoperative chest x-ray and CT scan of the brain were normal. Barium enema with air contrast, upper gastrointestinal series, and CT scan of the abdomen, done in May of 1982, were all normal; however, a postoperative abdominal CT scan revealed a 1 cm lesion in the dome of the right lobe of the liver and a 3 mm lesion adjacent to it. The head of the pancreas was enlarged with a 2 cm area of decreased attenuation.

Several forms of therapy were then tried:

1. The patient began a macrobiotic diet on August 7, 1982.

2. Beginning on August 18, 1982, he received a single course of palliative chemotherapy consisting of FAM (5-fluorouracil [5-FU], doxorubicin [Adriamycin], and mitomycin C), five treatments over five weeks at the Vince Lombardi Cancer Center of Georgetown University.

3. On September 23, 1982, he received a single dose of mouse monoclonal antibodies, which were develped by Dr. Hilary Koprowski of the Wistar Institue of the University of Pennsylvania, and given by Dr. Henry Sears, of American Oncologic Hospital in Philadelphia. Physicians at both the Vince Lombardi Cancer Center and the American Oncologic Hospital reviewed the biopsy slides and medical records and concurred with the diagnosis of metastatic adenocarcinoma of the pancreas.

The patient found the chemotherapy debilitating and felt it was not helping him; therefore, after the initial five-week course of chemotherapy the patient chose to discontinue all forms of conventional medical therapy. However, he remained on the macrobiotic diet.

An abdominal scan done on December 29, 1982, showed no enlargement of the hepatic metastasis. The pancreas was difficult to define owing to the almost total absence of retroperitoneal fat planes. On June 24, 1983, CT scan revealed no definite evidence of metastatic disease of the liver; furthermore, no mass could be defined in the pancreas. On December 21, 1983, the CT scan showed no measurable disease. As of this writing, nine years from his surgery, the patient is very active and in excellent health. He remains on the macrobiotic diet.

Of 250 patients with cancer in this patient's group who received mouse monoclonal antibodies, this is the only patient to survive (H. Koprowski, personal communication). It is therefore important that macrobiotics be considered as a possible reason for regression in this case. This remission is especially noteworthy, as pancreatic cancers are usually rapidly fatal.

Case B

This fifty-four year old white male was diagnosed as having malignant melanoma, Stage I, in 1973, which was widely excised, including auxillary and groin nodes. The patient had no further evidence of disease from 1973 until November, 1981, when a round lesion 1.5 cm in diameter developed 4 inches from the primary site on the right upper chest. The area was widely excised, and the lesion was determined to be a subcutaneous nodule of malignant melanoma consistent with metastatic growth. The patient began a one-year course of immunotherapy. In February, 1982, a suspicious-appearing spot was found on the primary site scar, which was again confirmed as melanoma and was again widley excised. In November, 1983, a routine follow-up chest x-ray revealed a spot on the right lung. On November 28, 1983, the patient underwent a thoracotomy and, at surgery, was found to have multiple tumor implants in all three lobes of the right lung, as well as on the diaphragm and chest wall in multiple areas. A wedge biopsy was taken of one of the diaphragmatic lesions, and the diagnosis of metastatic malignant melanoma was confirmed.

On January 3, 4, 5, and 6, 1984, the patient received a single four-day course of the BOLD regimen of palliative chemotherapy, consisting of bleomycin, DTIC, CCNU, and vincristine. Four weeks later the patient elected to discontinue all medical therapy and began macrobiotics. A chest x-ray approximately three weeks later showed a decrease in the size of the lesion compared to the previous chest x-ray of December 6, 1983. The chest x-ray also showed pleural diaphragmatic adhesions, which were doubtlessly due to scarring in the region of the biopsy. On March 27, 1985, no evidence of disease and no nodule could be seen on chest x-ray; an x-ray taken on September 9, 1985, duplicates these findings.

Now, nine years since his thoracotomy, and still adhering closely to macrobiotics, this patient reports experiencing the best health he can remember.

As with other cancers, spontaneous regression of melanoma is known to occur; however, the frequency is extremely rare.

Case C

This is a fifty-one year old white female who, in April of 1980, underwent a total abdominal hysterectomy and bilateral salpingo-oophorectomy at the age of forty for uterine tumor. Definitive diagnosis of the tumor was reached by light and electron microscopy, and it was determined to be an anaplastic, highly malignant endometrial stromal sarcoma. Bone scan and chest x-rays at this time were normal.

Postoperatively, the patient received palliative therapy in the form of 20 radiation treatments, a radium implant, and chemotherapy in the form of cytoxan and Megace.

By May, 1982, the patient was complaining increasingly of backache, and a bone scan revealed a compression fracture of L2. Chest x-rays taken on September 28, 1982, showed metastasis to the lungs as well as to the ninth thoracic and second lumbar vertebrae. At this time, the patient's chemotherapy was increased to include CCNU, doxorubicin (Adriamycin), 5-fluorouracil, and Megace. She also received an additional 10 radiation treatments. The patient was experiencing increasingly severe pain and could walk only with great difficulty. By January, 1983, the patient's x-rays revealed complete collapse of the body of L2, and the chest x-ray showed multiple pulmonary metastasis bilaterally.

In the same month, the patient sustained a paper cut injury to the thumb, which became infected, and she was hospitalized for intravenous antibiotic therapy in view of her degree of immunosuppression. She also received four units of packed cells as her hemoglobin level had dropped to 5.7 gm.

Upon discharge from the hospital, the patient was told that her chemotherapy would be continued at a lower dose. She elected to try an alternative form of therapy and, in February of 1983, began macrobiotics. The patient was unable to walk, was confined to a wheelchair, and was on high doses of narcotic analgesics for constant pain. Once the patient began macrobiotics, she discontinued all medical therapy, including all analgesics. Within one month of begining macrobiotics, the patient's pain had subsided. By March 27, 1983, the patient was able to walk without assistance. By February

18, 1985, a follow-up chest x-ray showed total regression of all the metastases except for one questionable lesion.

At present, eight years later, this patient is very active and in excellent health. She continues to follow a macrobiotic approach to her life.

Case D

D is a forty-four year old white male who, at the age of thirty-six, was admitted to the hospital on May 12, 1983, for a right colectomy with a preoperative diagnosis of adenocarcinoma of the ascending colon. The patient had involvement of the most proximal lymph node (Dukes C-1 classification). Preoperative liver-spleen scan was normal other than the minimal bone marrow uptake seen with anemia, which this patient had owing to chronic, severe rectal bleeding. At surgery, the liver and abdominal cavity were inspected carefully, and no metastases were found. The patient did not receive any postoperative chemotherapy or radiation therapy. This patient has a strong family history of carcinoma. His father died at age forty-six of carcinoma of the large bowel, as did his father's mother, at the age of thirty-two. His paternal grandmother's sister had three primary carcinomas — of the breast, uterus, and large bowel; she died from the colonic cancer.

On December 13, 1983, the patient had a follow-up liver-spleen scan, which revealed multiple filling defects. CT scan of the abdomen was then done, and it revealed multiple irregular focal lesions within the liver, compatible with multiple metastases. Hepatic angiography indicated that only the right lobe of the liver appeared to be involved. Therefore, the patient was transferred to the care of a specialist in Pittsburgh, in the hope of resecting the right lobe of the liver.

At an exploratory laparotomy, the right lobe was found to have multiple palpable metastatic lesions, several of which were visible grossly. As revealed by palpation, the left lobe had at least three sizable lesions. The remainder of the abdominal findings were normal. An extremely small true cut needle biopsy specimen was taken from the most accessible of the visible lesions. The surgeon stated that there was absolutely no doubt in his mind that this was a case of metastatic adenocarcinoma to the liver, and that he had taken the biopsy specimen for academic purposes only.

The pathology report stated that the specimen consisted of two fragments of soft, yellow tissue which were friable and measured 0.2 x 0.2 x 0.1 cm. in aggregate. No normal hepatic tissue was seen. Fibrosis and necrosis with calcifications were prominent. A small collection of nondiagositic epithelial cells was present on one end of the specimen.

The biopsy specimen was suspicious for, but not diagnostic of, carcinoma.

Postoperatively, as soon as food could be tolerated, the patient began macrobiotics and received no further medical therapy in any form. On June 29, 1984, the patient had a follow-up CT scan. This showed a decrease in size and perhaps also in the number of liver lesions. At least three of the lesions had become calcified. A further follow-up study on November 29, 1985, revealed a disappearance of some of the lesions; the remaining multiple hepatic metastases had become densely calcified.

As of this writing, eight years since surgery, the patient enjoys excellent health and remains on a macrobiotic diet.

For the purposes of this paper, it is unfortunate that the biopsy in this case was not diagnostic of metastatic adenocarcinoma; however, the case has been carefully reviewed by some of the leading pathologists in this country, and given the patient's history, the CT scans, and the observations of an experienced surgeon, in their opinion this case represents a case of regression of advanced metastatic adenocarcinoma of the colon.

Case E

This fifty-nine year old white male first came to medical attention when he complained of increasing abdominal discomfort and fullness over a period of six months. Palpation revealed a large, slightly tender tumor encompassing the entire right side of the abdomen. CT scan performed on March 9, 1983, showed a large multilobular, irregular mass within the abdomen, causing displacement of the urinary bladder to the left. The greatest transverse measurement of the mass was 16.5 cm, and it contained small loops of bowel within it. On fiberoptic sigmoidoscopy, the tumor was found to be causing extraluminal pressure and narrowing of the bowel.

On March 11, 1983, the patient underwent an exploratory laparotomy, at which time the tumor was found to be inoperable owing to the multiple loops of small bowel embedded within the tumor. Two biopsy specimens were taken.

Light microscopy of the specimen revealed multiple mitotic figures in most high power fields. Definitive diagnosis was reached through electron microscopy, and the tumor was determined to be a leiomyosarcoma; however, the possiblity that this tumor was a hemangiopericytoma could not be excluded.

On March 23, 1983, the patient elected to try macrobiotics. Between March 1983, and July 1983, the patient received four palliative courses of doxorubicin (Adriamycin) to a total dose of 560 mg. On July 29, 1983, the patient chose to discontinue all chemotherapy as he did not feel the chemotherapy was helping him. Earlier that month, on July 1, 1983, an abdominal CT scan showed a considerable decrease in the size of the mass to 10 cm at its maximum diameter, and a repeat CT scan, performed on May 1, 1985, showed no evidence of tumor.

After enjoying five to six years of good health with macrobiotics, the patient began to expand his diet considerably. Also in January, 1989, his life became more stressful. In July, 1989, his tumor recurred, and this time he was strongly advised to undergo chemotherapy. He experienced multiple complications and died in March, 1990.

Case F

F was a young person with a highly malignant, medically incurable cancer. The patient underwent surgery in an attempt to resect the tumor and also received chemotherapy and radiation. After only a few months, the tumor regrew to its original size. This time the patient turned to macrobiotics, experienced a rapid improvement, and was able to resume a normal active life. Serial CT scans revealed a steady decrease in the size of the tumor, until just over a year later the tumor was essentially gone.

Several months later the patient decided to travel widely, began eating many foods not regularly eaten in macrobiotics, and changed from gas to electric cooking. The patient became markedly symptomatic and a CT scan showed complete regrowth of the tumor. The tumor was again resected, and the patient attempted to cook macrobiotically again, but was unable to do so due to the severity of the symptoms. Several months later the patient succumbed to cancer and died.

While trying to locate cases of regression from advanced cancer for this study, I came across many anecdotal cases like the case of F in which the patient experienced complete remission of their cancer while on macrobiotics, only to go off the macrobiotic diet and have the cancer return and die from it. From the medical standpoint this case is extremely important in that the cancer disappeared while the patient was following the macrobiotic approach, but when she deviated widely (essentially stopped macrobiotics) the cancer regrew.

Discussion

Sometimes when I present these cases at a meeting, somebody will ask if these recoveries are simply due to spontaneous regression of cancer which has always been known to occur. Yes, it's true, spontaneous regression of cancer has been known to occur, but science has no idea why. Cases of spontaneous regression from cancer are extremely rare. To illustrate, the Institute of Noetic Sciences did a thorough search of the world literature from 1900 to 1987 (1) and found there to be less than 1000 cases of documented spontaneous regression from cancer. When one considers that approximately 20 percent of all deaths in the United States are from cancer, it is apparent just how rare spontaneous regression from cancer is. In another study, Everson and Cole (2,3) reviewed 176 cases of cancer that regressed without treatment. This study consisted of cases reported in the literature they researched from 1900 to 1964 and additional cases referred by other physicians. The criteria used by Everson and

Cole were not as strict as the criteria used for the cases reported here, since they included patients with partial as well as complete disappearance of tumors, and also cases in which the tumor decreased in size or disappeared in some areas of the body, while actually growing in other areas. Of the 176 cases reported, most did not live long: only 35 lived between 5 and 10 years, and in only 22 the regression lasted more than 10 years. Thus you can see just how rare it is for cancer to regress completely. Everson and Cole were unable to find any clear factors common to all the cases which could account for any of the regressions. The studies done by the Institute of Noetic Sciences and by Everson and Cole emphasize the extreme rarity of sustained regression from cancer, and thus the importance of the cases reported here. With this in mind, one would think that scientists would be keen to review any cases of spontaneous regression of cancer. All of the cases reported here have one major factor in common. All used macrobiotics. It is appropriate to question, therefore, the role which macrobiotics may have played in these regressions.

Some critics say the cases reported here are not worth considering because some of the patients recieved conventional therapy, such as chemotherapy. Therefore they cannot attribute any aspect of their recovery to macrobiotics. That would be a reasonable response if the conventional therapy received was known to be effective, and other patients had recovered from those cancers after receiving the same therapy. But the truth is, in all the cases described, the conventional therapy is known to be only palliative, that is, the therapy which was given is known to produce at best, a temporary decrease in the size of the tumor and a possible prolongation in life expectancy. Conventional therapy is known not to have resulted in any cases of sustained regression or recovery from any of these cancers.

The question arises, if macrobiotics played a significant role in the regression of these tumors, how and why does it work? Perhaps part of the reason lies in the observation that many of the components of the macrobiotic diet have been found to have either a strong or a possible antitumor effect (4,5). It would seem obvious this alone would make the dietary aspect of macrobiotics worth investigating as a possible benefit for cancer patients. For example, shiitake mushrooms, which are consumed frequently on the macrobiotic diet, have been shown to have a strong antitumor effect in mice. (6) Miso soup, eaten daily, has been found to significantly reduce the frequency of stomach cancer in Japan. (7) Certain sea vegetables may have an antitumor effect in mice (8) and rats.(9) Sea vegetables may also inhibit the intestinal absorption of radioactive products and possibly help decontaminate the body after exposure to radioactive materials. Investigators have reported sea vegetables contain a polysaccharide that selectively binds radioactive strontium and helps eliminate it from the body. (10, 11) How many other foods commonly eaten in macrobiotics do you think might be found to have antitumor effects, or other effects which might be beneficial to the body if they were apapropriately investigated?

In addition, the macrobiotic diet avoids chemically treated, highly processed, and heavily salted foods. It is very low in fats (most diets for seriously ill patients have about 8 to 12 percent fat which is known to improve the prognosis in some forms of cancer [12, 13, 14]). The macrobiotic diet is high in fiber and complex carbohydrates, high in folic acid, selenium, and vitamins A and C. Many of the component foods are known to decrease cancer risk; therefore, the diet may both reduce a person's chances of developing cancer and possibly enhance regression of established cancers.

For various reasons, macrobiotics has not been accepted by the medical community. Some of the lack of acceptance may result from a serious misunderstanding about the nature of this alternative approach to healing. Many of the original analyses of macrobiotics were based on misinterpretations of the teachings of macrobiotics which resulted in a few followers of macrobiotics developing serious and even fatal vitamin deficiencies. Unfortunately, this view that macrobiotics is nutritionally unsound has persisted in the medical community. I have seen it turn into tragic results on several occassions when patients with advanced cancer who had been doing well with macrobiotics went back to their doctors and were advised to add various foods to their diet, usually milk, meat and poultry. If the patient chose to follow this advice and added these foods to their macrobiotic diet, they created a severe imbalance. I have seen many patients who were doing extremely well deteriorate rapidly and die after making such changes.

Several careful investigations have recently been done of macrobiotic diets and have shown, not only are macrobiotic diets nutritionally sound, but they are also consistent with the guidelines issued by the National Cancer Institute and the American Cancer Society. They emphasize whole grains, fresh vegetables and fruits, and limit fatty animal products, sugars, and artificial additives. As Dr. Martha Cottrell has eloquently discussed in her book, *AIDS, Macrobiotics and Natural Immunity* written in conjunction with Michio Kushi and Mark Mead, dietary fats, simple sugars, cow's milk proteins, and food additives (approximately 3,000 of which are found in our food supply, including pesticides, herbicides, preservatives, colorings, flavorings, texturizers, and others), may weaken the immune system. Also they may be associated with an increased risk of developing not only cancer, but also heart disease, diabetes, obesity, renal failure, gastrointestinal diseases, and allergies. Dr. Cottrell goes on to explain that some foods included in the macrobiotic diet (for example, soy products: high in lecithin, seaweeds: rich in minerals, and green leafy vegetables: high in vitamin C, beta-carotene, and calcium) may strengthen the immune system (15, 16, 17, 18, 19, 20, 21, 22).

It is important to understand that macrobiotics is not an outgrowth of dietary advice based on current scientific knowledge, but rather an ancient traditional understanding of living in harmony with nature and with every aspect of our lives. A major goal of macrobiotics is to give an understanding of the flow of energy in all things including food. When we have that understanding of the energy in food and in our environment, then we can learn to eat in a way that creates balance. Then we can create the physical, emotional and spiritual health to fulfill our dreams and goals in life. The entire focus of Oriental healing is to create higher states of health. Oriental experts have addressed such questions as what foods improve mental clarity and focus, improve sleep, and improve physical endurance. Thus, macrobiotics evolved to create health, rather than to cure illness. When illness did occur, Orientals believed if properly nourished and cared for, and with careful attention to positive thinking, the body would heal itself. The present macrobiotic approach to healing illness evolved from the compassion and dedication that people like Michio Kushi and other macrobiotic counsellors had for those who were suffering from serious illnesses. Through their understanding of the flow of energy, especially in food, they assist sick people to regenerate and recover from their illnesses.

The question arises for the person with a serious illness, particularly a rapidly fatal illness, what are the chances that macrobiotics will help, and will this approach give the highest chance of recovery? No one knows the answers to these and similar questions, such as which form of unconventional therapy offers the greatest chance of recovery? Many Americans have asked to have these questions addressed, so Congress commissioned the Office of Technology and Assessment [OTA], to investigate unconventional treatments used by cancer patients. It is difficult to believe that a government agency which was asked to perform a task that could affect the lives of one in five Americans (one in five Americans die from cancer), would do such a poor job. Tragically, in my view, they did an appalling job. After spending hundreds of thousands of tax dollars, OTA did not interview one single cancer patient who had used an unconventional therapy. In reviewing macrobiotics, the report dwelt on the areas which seemed unscientific to them and skimmed over the cases which I and others had documented, stating that the cases were merely retrospective (cases that had already recovered, as opposed to prospective). Never did they ask to review any of the cases. Why do they have so little interest in these cases, and why are they so quick to criticize the work as retrospective? They have not been able to demonstrate one case of sustained regression from any of these cancers using any form of conventional medicine, despite the billions of dollars spent on research. Even more tragic, this report failed to result in appropriate research to determine which form of therapy, conventional or unconventional, yields the highest chance of recovery for different cancers.

How do I attempt to answer these difficult questions? First, I remind patients that no one knows the answer. Patients must look within themselves, and take full responsibility for making their own decisions. Second, I share with them the characteristics I have noticed in people who have done well. Briefly they include: (a) patients have to hold to their diet absolutely accurately; (b) ideally someone who cares about the patient does some of the cooking for them; (c) patients must have a profound desire to live and be open to change and do whatever is necessary to recover; (d) patients need to have a willingness to accept responsibility for having created their illness and accept the responsibility for curing their illness; (e) probably of greatest importance, patients need strong family support, both by cooking and eating macrobiotically with them. This develops an understanding of macrobiotics and creates a team commitment for the challenges being faced. If you would like to know more about these aspects of recovery, then you might like to read an article I wrote entitled "Macrobiotics: An Approach to Health, Happiness and Harmony" in the book *Doctors Look at Macrobiotics.*

It is apparent, therefore, that recovery from advanced cancer using macrobiotics requires enormous commitment and willingness to change, both by the patient and by the patient's family. Patients with advanced cancer who are trying to recover using macrobiotics must recognize they are hoping for a miracle. The good news is that some people have succeeded. In my experience, the majority of people with advanced cancer who try macrobiotics do not succeed, mainly because of a lack of family support and the terrible isolation which patients experience as they attempt to cook for themselves and eat alone. This emphasizes the importance that any attempts by the scientific community to investigate the efficacy of macrobiotics must be done in close cooperation with the macrobiotic community.

Some patients ask, is it wise to use macrobiotics instead of conventional medicine? In view of the small number of people who have recovered using macrobiotics, if conventional therapy offers any true possibility of curing the disease, in my opinion the patient is wise to use both macrobiotics and conventional therapy. On the other hand, if conventional therapy offers no possibility of curing the disease, the patient is probably better off with macrobiotics alone. Conventional therapy often has a very debilitating effect on the immune system and seems to decrease the effectiveness of macrobiotics.

In addition to cases of advanced cancer that have recovered using macrobiotics, I have come across a very wide range of illnesses ranging from relatively benign problems like premenstrual tension and migraine headaches, to extremely serious medically incurable illnesses that were either dramatically improved or cured using macrobiotics. The list of medically incurable illnesses includes diseases such as advanced rhuematoid arthritis, myasthenia gravis, advanced diabetes and diabetic retinopathy, renal failure, multiple sclerosis, to name just a few. When people changed to a macrobiotic way of life, they seemed to experience improvements in every area of their life, particularly in overall health, vitality, mental clarity and psychological well being, as well as improved emotional stability and serenity.

In conclusion, macrobiotics offers the possibility of improved health, vitality and well-being for anyone who tries it. Macrobiotics also offers hope for the hopeless.

Acknowledgments

I would like to express my sincere appreciation to the following persons: Dr. Joseph Horstman, Chief of Pathology, Holy Redeemer Hospital, for reading the slides and discussing the appropriateness of the cases with me; Dr. John Faulkner, Department of Radiology, Holy Redeemer Hospital, for reviewing the x-rays: David Westwater, without whose tireless help I would never have been able to contact all the patients; Professor Yoshio Watanabe, for invaluable comments and inspiration; and Michio Kushi, Denny Waxman, Geraldine Walker and all the macrobiotic counselors whose encouragement and support made this paper possible.

References

1. O'Reagan, B.: *Healing, remission and miracle cures.* Special report, Washington Committee of the Institute of Noetic Sciences, American University, December 5, 1986. © 1987, The Institute of Noetic Sciences.

2. Everson, T.C., and Cole, W.H.: *Spontaneous Regression of Cancer.* Philadelphia, W.B. Saunders Company, 1966.

3. Cole, W.H.: "Efforts to explain spontaneous regression of cancer." *J Surg. Oncol.* 17:201-209, 1981.

4. Akizuki, T.: "How we survived Nagasaki." *East-West J.*, December 1980, pp.10-12.

5. Akizuki, T.: *Nagasaki 1945.* London, Quartet Books, 1981.

6. Chihara, G., Hamuro, J., Maeda, Y.Y., et al.: "Fractionation and purification of polysaccharides with marked anti-tumor activity, especially lentinan, from *Lentinus edodes* (Berk.) Sing. (an edible mushroom)." *Cancer Res.* 30:2776-2781, 1970.

7. Hirayama, T.: "Relationship of soybean paste soup intake to gastric cancer risk," *J. Nutr. Cancer* 3:223-233, 1982.

8. Yamamoto, I. , Nagumo, T., Yagi, K, et al.: "Antitumor effects of seaweeds. I. Antitumor effect of extracts from Sargassum and Laminaria." *Jpn. J. Exp. Med.*, 44: 543-546, 1974.

9. Teas, J., Harbison, M.L., and Gelman, R.S.: "Dietary seaweed (Lamianria) and mammary carcinogenesis in rats." *Cancer Res.* 44:2758-2761, 1984.

10. Skoryna, S.C., et al.: "Studies of the inhibition of intestinal absorption of radioactive strontium." *Can. Med. Assoc. J.* 91:285-288, 1964.

11. Tanaka, Y., Waldron-Edward, D., and Skoryna, S.C.: "Studies on inhibition of intestinal absorption of radioactive strontium." *Can. Med. Assoc. J.* 99:169-175, 1968.

12. Cruse, P., Lewin, M.R., and Clark, C.G.: "Dietary cholesterol deprivation improves survival rates and reduces incidence of metastatic colon cancer in dimethylhydrazine-pretreated rats." *Gut* 23:594-599, 1982.

13. Tartter, P.I., Papatestas, A.E., Ioannovich, J., et al.: "Cholesterol and obesity as prognostic factors in breast cancer." *Cancer* 47:2222-2227, 1981.

14. Willett, W.C., Stampfer, M.J., Colditz, G.A., et al: "Dietary fat and the risk of breast cancer." *N. Engl. J. Med.* 316:22-28, 1987.

15. Kushi, Michio and Cottrell, Martha, M.D.: *AIDS, Macrobiotics and Natural Immunity,* Tokyo and New York, Japan Publications, 1990.

16. Talbott, M., Miller, L.T., Kerkvliet, N.I.: "Pyridoxine supplementation: Effect on lymphocyte responses in elderly persons." *Am. J. Clin. Nutr.* 46:659-664, 1987.

17. Panush, R.S., and Delafuente, J.C.: "Vitamins and immunocompetence." *World Rev. Nutr. Diet.* 45:97-132, 1985.

18. Alexander, M., Newmark, H., Miller, R.G., et al.: "Oral beta-carotene can increase the number of OKT4+ cells in human blood." *Immunol.* Lett. 9:221-224, 1985.

19. Menkes, M.S, Constock, G.W., Vuillemier, J.P., et al.: "Serum beta-carotene, vitamins A and E, selenium, and the risk of lung cancer." *N. Engl. J. Med.* 315:1250-1254, 1986.

20. Anderson, R.: The immunostimulatory, anti-inflammatory and anti-allergic properties of ascorbate." *Adv. Nutr. Res.* 6:19-45, 1984.

21. Tanaka, J., Fujiwara, H., and Torisu, M.: "Vitamin E and immune resonse. I. Enhancement of helper T cell activity by dietary supplementation of vitamin E in mice." *Immunolog* 38:727-734, 1979.

22. Good, R.A., and Lorenz, E.: "Nutrition, immunity, aging, and cancer: Zinc and immunocompetence." *Nutr. Rev.* 46:62-67, 1988.

Dr. Newbold received her medical degree from the University of Edinburgh, Scotland, in 1974 and went on to specialize in emergency medicine, becoming a fellow of the American College of Emergency Physicians in 1984.

Part IV
Appendixes

Appendix I
Principles and Laws of the Infinite Universe

Seven Universal Principles
1. Everything is a differentiation of one Infinity.
2. Everything changes.
3. All antagonisms are complementary.
4. There is nothing identical to anything else.
5. What has a front (i.e., a visible side) has a back (i.e., an invisible side).
6. The bigger the front, the bigger the back.
7. What has a beginning has an end.

Twelve Laws of Change
1. One Infinity manifests itself in complementary and antagonistic tendencies, yin and yang, in its endless change.
2. Yin and yang are manifested continuously from the eternal movement of one infinite universe.
3. Yin represents centrifugality. Yang represents centripetality. Yin and yang together produce energy and all phenomena.
4. Yin attracts yang. Yang attracts yin.
5. Yin repels yin. Yang repels yang.
6. Yin and yang combined in varying proportions produce different phenomena. The attraction and repulsion between phenomena is proportional to the difference of the yin and yang forces within them.

7. All phenomena are ephemeral, constantly changing their constitution of yin and yang forces; yin changes into yang, yang changes into yin.

8. Nothing is solely yin or solely yang. Everything is composed of both tendencies in varying degrees.

9. There is nothing neutral. Either yin or yang is predominant in every phenomenon.

10. Large yin attracts small yin. Large yang attracts small yang.

11. Extreme yin produces yang, and extreme yang produces yin.

12. All physical manifestations are yang at the center and yin at the surface.

Appendix II
Research on Cancer and Diet Related to Macrobiotics

Within the last several years, the macrobiotic approach to cancer has begun to attract increasing scientific interest. Some of these studies have begun to be published. Others are still in progress. Those specifically relating to cancer or cancer risk factors are summarized below:

A. Breast Cancer

Vegetarian women appear to be at less risk of developing breast cancer, researchers at New England Medical Center in Boston reported in 1981. The scientists found that vegetarian women process estrogen differently from other women and eliminate it more quickly from their bodies. The study involved 45 pre- and post-menopausal women, about half of whom were vegetarian and half non-vegetarian. The women consumed about the same number of total calories. Although the vegetarian women took in only one third as much animal protein and animal fat, they excreted two to three times as much estrogen. High levels of estrogen have been associated with the development of breast cancer. "The difference in estrogen metabolism may explain the lower incidence of breast cancer in vegetarian women," the study concluded.

Source: B.R. Goldin et al., "Effect of Diet on Excretion of Estrogens in Pre- and Post-menopausal Incidence of Breast Cancer in Vegetarian Women," Cancer Research 41: 3771-73.

Note: The vegetarian participants (subjects) were people on a macrobiotic diet, though the report calls them "vegetarian."

B. Macrobiotic vs. Conventional Treatment

In 1984, a team of researchers at medical schools and hospitals in Boston, headed by Dr. Robert Lerman, Director of Clinical Nutrition at University Hospital, announced plans to evaluate several hundred cancer patients who had tried the macrobiotic dietary approach and match them with controls from the Eastern Cooperative Oncology Group tumor registry at the Dana-Farber Cancer Institute in Boston. Data has been gathered, but final results have not as yet been published.

C. Kaposi's Sarcoma

In 1984, immunologists in New York and Boston began to monitor the blood samples and immune functions of ten men with Kaposi's sarcoma (a malignancy associated with AIDS) who had begun the macrobiotic dietary approach. Reports of their ongoing progress appeared in *The Lancet* (2:223, July 27, 1985) and in a paper presented at the International AIDS Conference in Paris, France, 1986 entitled "Patients with Kaposi's Sarcoma Who Opt for Alternative Therapy."

D. Cancer and General Health

In 1986, Dr. Peter Gruner, Director of Oncology at St. Mary's Hospital in Montreal, Canada, launched a study of approximately thirty individuals on macrobiotic diets to find if there were significant differences between their levels of health and those of the general population. Gruner subjected the participants, who had been practicing a macrobiotic diet for anywhere from nine months to fourteen years, to a battery of physiological tests. "I am impressed positively about it," he told *The Gazette*, a Montreal daily newspaper. "Everything measured normal in their blood; blood pressure was normal; there were no calcium, B-12 or iron deficiencies. (There) was a surprisingly low blood cholesterol level, far and away the best cholesterol measure I have ever seen."

Source: Harriet Fels, "Testing the Macrobiotic Miracle," The Living Section, *The Gazette*, Montreal, Canada, Nov. 20, 1987.

E. Cancer Risk Factors

After studying the blood values of twenty macrobiotic men, J. P. Deslypere, M.D., a research team member from the Academic field of the Ghent University in Belgium, concluded, "In the field of cardiovascular and cancer risk factors this kind of blood is very favorable. It's ideal, we couldn't do better; that's what we're dreaming of. It's really fantastic, like children, whose blood vessels are still completely open and whole. This is a very important matter, deserving our full attention."

Source: *The World of Science*, Ghent, Belgium, Fall, 1983.

F. Radiation Sickness

In August, 1945, at the time of the atomic bombing of Japan, Tatsuichiro Akizuki, M.D., was director of the Department of Internal Medicine at St. Francis's Hospital in Nagasaki. Most patients in the hospital, located one mile from the epicenter of the blast, survived the initial effects of the bomb but soon after came down with symptoms of radiation sickness from the fallout that had been released.

Dr. Akizuki fed his staff and patients a strict macrobiotic diet of brown rice, miso and tamari soy sauce soup, wakame and other seaweeds, Hokkaido pumpkin, and sea salt and prohibited the consumption of sugar and sweets. As a result, he saved everyone in his hospital, while many other survivors in the city perished from radiation sickness.

Sources: Tatsuichiro Akizuki, M.D., "How We Survived Nagasaki," *East West Journal,* December, 1980, pp. 10-12, and Tatsuichiro Akizuki, M.D., *Nagasaki 1945,* London: Quartet Books, 1981.

Note: Dr. Akizuki is still living in Nagasaki where he is director of St. Francis' Hospital and chairman of the Nagasaki Hibakusha (atomic bomb survivors) organization.

G. Cancer-Prevention

The standard macrobiotic dietary approach emphasizes whole grains and vegetables, including foods rich in vitamins A and C in the daily diet and cruciferous vegetables associated with the prevention of some forms of cancer. Altogether grains account for about 50 percent of total daily food intake by volume, and a wide variety of vegetables, prepared in different ways, make up usually from 25-30 percent. Beans, seeds, and nuts are also eaten regularly, and for those who choose to eat animal quality food, white-meat fish or seafood is taken, usually in moderate volume several times a week. The scientific and medical community have recently devoted considerable attention to these foods, so we will not list these findings in detail.

Besides grains, vegetables, beans, seeds and nuts, and fish and seafood, however, there are a number of specific foods emphasized in the standard macrobiotic dietary approach that have been associated with protecting against cancer. These include:

Miso Soup

In 1981, Japan's National Cancer Center reported that people who eat miso soup daily are 33 percent less likely to contract stomach cancer and have 19 percent less cancer at other sites than those who never eat miso soup.

Source: T. Hirayama, "Relationship of Soybean Paste Soup Intake to Gastric Cancer Risk," *Nutrition and Cancer* 3: 223-33.

Note: Miso soup is eaten usually once or twice a day in most macrobiotic homes in the United States. In addition to soup, miso is used to make sauces, dressings, dips, and spreads and is used occasionally in place of salt as a seasoning for grains, beans, or vegetables.

Sea Vegetables

In a 1984 experiment at the Harvard School of Public Health, laboratory animals fed a control diet with 5 percent Halies (kombu), a brown sea vegetable, developed induced mammary cancer later than animals not fed seaweed. "Seaweed has shown consistent antitumor activity in several *in vivo* animal tests," the researcher concluded. "In extrapolating these results to the Japanese population seaweed may be an important factor in explaining the low rates of certain cancers in Japan."

Source: J. Teas, M.L. Harbison, and R.S. Gelman, "Dietary Seaweed [*Laminaria*] and Mammary Carcinogensis in Rats," *Cancer Research* 44: 2758-61.

In 1974, Japanese researchers reported that several varieties of kombu and mojaban, common sea vegetables eaten in Asia, were effective in the treatment of tumors in laboratory experiments. In three of four samples tested, inhibition rates in mice with implanted sarcomas ranged from 89 to 95 percent. The researchers reported that "the tumor underwent complete regression in more than half of the mice of each treated group." Similar experiments on mice with leukemia showed promising results.

Source: I. Yamamoto et al., "Antitumor Effect of Seaweeds," *Japanese Journal of Experimental Medicine* 44: 543-46.

In 1968, Canadian scientists at the Gastro-Intestinal Research Laboratory at McGill University in Montreal, Canada designed an experiment to evaluate whether a food substance could help counteract the effects of nuclear radiation which has been associated with a increase in leukemia, bone cancer, and other malignancies. The researchers reported that sea vegetables contained a polysaccharide substance that selectively bound radioactive strontium and helped eliminate it from the body. In laboratory experiments, sodium alginate prepared from kelp, kombu, and other brown seaweeds off the Atlantic and Pacific coasts was introduced along with strontium and calcium into rats. The reduction of radioactive particles in bone uptake, measured in the femur, reached as high as 80 percent, with little interference with calcium absorption. "The evaluation of biological activity of different marine algae is important because of their practical significance in preventing absorption of radioactive products of atomic fission as well as in their use as possible natural decontaminars."

Source: Y. Tanaka et al., "Studies on Inhibition of Intestinal Absorption of Radio-Active Strontium," *Canadian Medical Association Journal* 99: 169-775, 1968. See also an earlier study by S.C. Skoryna et al., "Studies on Inhibition of Intestinal Absorption of Radioactive Strontium," *Canadian Medical Association Journal* 91: 285-88, 1964.

Note: Kombu and other seaweeds (sea vegetables) are an important part of the Standard Macrobiotic Dietary approach, accounting for about 5 percent of daily food intake by volume. In addition to being added to soup, seaweed is often prepared as a small side dish or a small piece of seaweed is cooked with grain or beans to provide additional minerals and vitamins. The Kushi Foundation cooperated with the Harvard School of Public Health in obtaining seaweed for their study.

Tofu

In 1971, in an epidemiological study involving several foods, a Japanese cancer researcher reported that people who regularly ate soybean curd (tofu) were at less risk for stomach cancer than those who did not.

Source: T. Hirayama, "Epidemiology of Stomach Cancer," in T. Murakami (ed.), *Early Gastric Cancer. Gann Monograph on Cancer Research*, 11 (Tokyo: University of Tokyo Press, pp. 3-19).

Note: The macrobiotic community helped introduce tofu to America, and it is now available in many supermarkets as well as natural foods stores and is enjoyed by many people. In most macrobiotic homes, tofu is eaten several times a week, prepared in various ways.

Shiitake Mushroom

In 1970, Japanese scientists at the National Cancer Center Research Institute reported that shiitake mushrooms had a strong anti-tumor effect. In experiments with mice, polysaccharide preparations from various natural sources, including the shiitake mushroom commonly available in Tokyo markets, markedly inhibited the growth of induced sarcomas resulting in "almost complete regression of tumors with no sign of toxicity."

Source: G. Chihara, et al., "Fractionation and Purification of the Polysaccharides with Marked Antitumor Activity, Especially Lentinan," from *Lentinus edodes* (Berk.) Sing. (An Edible Mushroom)," *Cancer Research* 30: 2776-81.

Note: Shiitake mushrooms are commonly used in macrobiotic households in soups, salads, and vegetable dishes, and they are occasionally prepared in a tea.

Dairy Food

Women with breast cancer tend to consume considerably more dairy food than healthy women the same age, according to a 1989 report in the *Journal of the National Cancer Institute*. In Italy, medical researchers compared 250 breast cancer patients in the northwest province of Vercelli with 499 normal women and found that the higher fat and protein intake typical of the breast cancer group was due entirely to higher consumption of meat and dairy food, especially milk, high-fat cheese, and butter.

Source: *Science News*, Feb. 18, 1989.

Note: Dairy foods are customarily avoided in the macrobiotic way of eating.

Appendix III
Dietary Goals and
Recommendations

Dietary Goals for the United States

In 1977, the U.S. Senate Select Committee on Nutrition and Human Needs issued *Dietary Goals for the United States*, a landmark report on the nation's way of eating, health, and future direction. The Senate findings, also known as the McGovern Report after its chairman, George McGovern, concluded:

> During this century, the composition of the average diet in the United States has changed radically. Complex carbohydrates — fruit, vegetables, and grain products — which were the mainstay of the diet, now play a minority role. At the same time, fat and sugar consumption have risen to the point where these two dietary elements along now comprise at least 60 percent of the total calorie intake, up from 50 percent in the early 1900s.

> In the view of doctors and nutritionists consulted by the Select Committee, these and other changes in the diet amount to a wave of malnutrition — of both over- and under-consumption — that may be as profoundly damaging to the Nation's health as the widespread contagious diseases of the early part of this century. The over-consumption of fat, generally, and saturated fat in particular, as well as cholesterol, sugar, salt, and alcohol

have been related to six of the leading causes of death: Heart disease, cancer, cerebrovascular diseases, diabetes, arteriosclerosis, and cirrhosis of the liver.

United States Dietary Goals:
1. Increase carbohydrate consumption to account for 55 to 66 percent of the energy (caloric) intake.
2. Reduce the overall fat consumption from approximately 40 to 30 percent of energy intake.
3. Reduce saturated fat consumption to account for about 10 percent of total energy intake; and balance with polyunsaturated and monounsaturated fats, which should account for about 10 percent of energy intake each.
4. Reduce cholesterol consumption to about 300 mg. a day.
5. Reduce sugar consumption by almost 40 percent to account for about 15 percent of total energy intake.
6. Reduce salt consumption by about 50 to 85 percent to approximately 3 grams a day.

Sources for current diet: *Changes in Nutrients in the U.S. Diet Caused by Alterations in Food Intake Patterns*. B. Friend. Agricultural Research Service. U.S. Department of Agriculture, 1974. Proportions of saturated versus unsaturated fats based on unpublished Agricultural Research Service data.

The Goals Suggest the Following Changes in Food Selection and Preparation:
1. Increase consumption of fruits and vegetables and whole grains.
2. Decrease consumption of meat and increase consumption of poultry and fish.
3. Decrease consumption of foods high in fat and partially substitute polyunsaturated fat for saturated fat.
4. Substitute non-fat milk for whole milk.
5. Decrease consumption of butterfat, eggs, and other high cholesterol sources.
6. Decrease consumption of sugar and foods that are high in

sugar content.
7. Decrease consumption of salt and food high in salt content.

Source: *Dietary Goals for the United States*, Senate Select Committee on Nutrition and Human Needs (Washington, D.C.: Government Printing Office, 1977).

The Surgeon General's Report

In 1979, the U.S. Surgeon General issued *Healthy People*, a report of the nation's health that suggested degenerative disease could be relieved as well as prevented by dietary means and called for substantial increases in consumption of whole grains, vegetables, and fresh fruit and reductions in meat, eggs, dairy food, sugar, and other processed foods. The report states in part:

> A good case can be made for the role of high intake of cholesterol and saturated fat, usually of animal origin, in producing high blood cholesterol levels which are associated with atherosclerosis and cardiovascular diseases. Animal studies have shown that reducing serum cholesterol can slow down and even reverse the atherosclerotic process.

> And, in man, certain studies have shown that people in countries where diets are low in saturated fats and cholesterol have lower average serum cholesterol levels and fewer heart attacks; and that Americans who habitually eat less fat-rich diets (vegetarians and Seventh-Day Adventists, for example) have less heart disease than other Americans. Other observations in man suggest the possibility that certain types of atherosclerosis may be reversed by cholesterol-lowering diets.

> Healthy Nutrition: Individual nutritional requirement variations make exact dietary standards impossible to establish. Variations also occur in the same person a different times — during pregnancy with aging, during acute or chronic illness, or with changes in physical activity.

But given what is already known or strongly suspected about the relationship between diet and disease, Americans would probably be healthier, as a whole if they consumed:

- only sufficient calories to meet body needs and maintain desirable weight (fewer calories if overweight);
- less saturated fat and cholesterol;
- less salt;
- less sugar;
- relatively more complex carbohydrates such as whole grains, cereals, fruits and vegetables; and
- relatively more fish, poultry, legumes (e.g., beans, peas, peanuts) and less red meat.

The processing of our food also makes a difference. The American food supply has changed so that more than half of our diet now consists of processed foods rather than fresh agricultural produce. Increased attention therefore also needs to be paid to the nutritional qualities of processed food.

Source: *Healthy People: The Surgeon General's Report on Health Promotion and Disease Prevention* (Washington, D.C.: Government Printing Office, 1979).

The National Academy of Sciences' Report on Cancer and Diet

In 1982, the National Academy of Sciences issued *Diet, Nutrition and Cancer*, a 472-page report to the National Cancer Institute, in which the modern diet was associated with a majority of common cancers, especially malignancies of the stomach, colon, breast, endometrium, and lung. The panel reviewed hundreds of current medical studies associating long-term eating patterns and estimated that diet is responsible for 30 percent to 40 percent of cancers in men and 60 percent of cancers in women.

Interim Dietary Guidelines: It is not now possible, and may

never be possible, to specify a diet that would protect everyone against all forms of cancer. Nevertheless, the committee believes that it is possible on the basis of current evidence to formulate interim dietary guidelines that are both consistent with good nutritional practices and likely to reduce the risk of cancer. These guidelines are meant to be applied in their entirety to obtain maximal benefit.

1. There is sufficient evidence that high fat consumption is linked to increased incidence of certain cancers (notably breast and colon cancer) and that low fat intake is associated with a lower incidence of these cancers. The committee recommends that the consumption of both saturated and unsaturated fats be reduced in the average U.S. diet. An appropriate and practical target is to reduce the intake of fat from its present level (approximately 40 percent) to 30 percent of total calories in the diet. The scientific data do not provide a strong basis for establishing fat intake at precisely 30 percent of total calories. Indeed, the data could be used to justify an even greater reduction. However, in the judgment of the committee, the suggested reduction (i.e., one-quarter of the fat intake) is a moderate and practical target, and is likely to be beneficial.

2. The committee emphasizes the importance of including fruits, vegetables, and whole grain cereal products in the daily diet. In epidemilogical studies, frequent consumption of these foods has been inversely correlated with the incidence of various cancers. Results of laboratory experiments have supported these findings in tests of individual nutritive and nonnutritive constituents of fruits (especially citrus fruits) and vegetables (especially carotene-rich and cruciferous vegetables).

These recommendations apply only to foods as sources of nutrients — not to dietary supplements of individual nutrients. The vast literature examined in this report focuses on the relationship between the consumption of foods and the incidence of cancer in human populations. In contrast, there is very little information of the effects of various levels of individual nutrients on the risk of cancer in humans. Therefore, the committee is unable to predict the health effects of high and potentially toxic doses of isolated nutrients consumed in the form of supplements.

3. In some parts of the world, especially China, Japan, and Iceland, populations that frequently consumed salt-cured (including salt-pickled) or smoked foods have a greater incidence of cancers at some sites, especially the esophagus and the stomach. In addition, some methods of smoking and pickling foods seem to produce higher levels of polycyclic aromatic hydrocarbons and N-nitroso compounds. These compounds cause mutations in bacteria and cancer in animals and are suspected of being carcinogenic in humans. Therefore, the committee recommends that the consumption of food preserved by salt-curing (including salt-pickling) or smoking be minimized.

4. Certain non-nutritive constituents of foods, whether naturally occurring or introduced inadvertently (as contaminants) during production, processing, and storage, pose a potential risk of cancer to humans. The committee recommends that efforts continue to be made to minimize contamination of foods with carcinogens from any source. Where such contaminants are unavoidable, permissible levels should continue to be established and the food supply monitored to assure that such levels are not exceeded. Furthermore, intentional additives (direct and indirect) should continue to be evaluated for carcinogenic activity before they are approved for use in the food supply.

5. The committee suggests that further efforts be made to identify mutagens in food and to expedite testing for their carcinogenicity. Where feasible and prudent, mutagens should be removed or their concentration minimized when this can be accomplished without jeopardizing the nutritive value of foods or introducing other potentially hazardous substances into the diet.

6. Excessive consumption of alcoholic beverages, particularly combined with cigarette smoking, has been associated with an increased risk of cancer of the upper gastrointestinal and respiratory tracts. Consumption of alcohol is also associated with other adverse health effects. Thus, the committee recommends that if alcoholic beverages are consumed, it be done in moderation.

Further Excerpts: Just as it was once difficult for investigators to recognize that a symptom complex could be caused by the lack of a nutrient, until recently has it been difficult for scientists to recognize that certain pathological conditions might result from an abundant and apparently normal diet . . .

Technological advances in recent years have led to changes in the methods of food processing, a greater assortment of food products, and as a result, changes in the consumption patterns of the U.S. population. The impact of these modifications on human health, especially the potential adverse effects of food additives and contaminants, has drawn considerable attention from the news media and the public. Advances in technology have resulted in an increased use of industrial chemicals, thereby increasing the potential for chemical contamination of drinking water and food supplies. The use of processed foods and, consequently, of additives, has also increased substantially during the past four decades . . . More than 55 percent of the food consumed in the United States today has been processed to some degree before distribution to the consumer . . .

The dietary changes now under way appear to be reducing our dependence on foods from animal sources. It is likely that there will be continued reduction in fats from animal sources and an increasing dependence on vegetable and other plant products for protein supplies. Hence, diets may contain increasing amounts of vegetables products, some of which may be protective against cancer . . .

Source: *Diet, Nutrition and Cancer* (Washington, D.C.: National Academy of Sciences, 1982).

American Cancer Society Dietary Guidelines

In 1984, the American Cancer Society issued dietary guidelines for the first time in respect to the cause and prevention of cancer.

> ... There is now good reason to suspect that dietary habits contribute to human cancer, but it is important to understand that the interpretation of both human population (epidemiologic) and laboratory data is very complex, and as yet does not allow clear-cut conclusions . . . Foods may have constituents that cause or promote cancer on the one hand or protect against it on the other. No concrete dietary advice can be given that will guarantee prevention of any specific human cancer. The American Cancer Society nonetheless believes that there is sufficient inferential information to make a series of interim recommendations about nutrition that, in the judgment of experts, are likely to provide some measure of reducing cancer risk . . .

Recommendations:
1. Avoid obesity.
2. Cut down on total fat intake.
3. Eat more high fiber foods, such as whole grain cereals, fruits and vegetables.
4. Include foods rich in vitamins A and C in the daily diet.
5. Include cruciferous vegetables, such as cabbage, broccoli, Brussels sprouts, kohlrabi, and cauliflower in the diet.
6. Be moderate in consumption of alcoholic beverages.
7. Be moderate in consumption of salt-cured, smoked, and nitrite-cured foods.

Source: *Nutrition and Cancer: Cause and Prevention* (New York: American Cancer Society, 1984).

Appendix IV
Macrobiotic Resources
and Recommended Reading

East West Foundation

The East West Foundation is a nonprofit, educational foundation founded by Michio and Aveline Kushi in 1973 devoted to informing the public about the relation of diet and degenerative disease and promoting better communication between East and West, North and South. Over the years, the East West Foundation has sponsored many conferences and symposia on cancer and diet, cooperated in medical and scientific research, and published case history reports and other study materials. The East West Foundation is presently coordinated out of the international One Peaceful World office in Becket, Massachusetts (see below).

One Peaceful World

One Peaceful World is an international information network and friendship society of individuals, families, educational centers, organic farmers, teachers and parents, authors and artists, publishers and business people, and others devoted to the realization of one healthy, peaceful world. Activities include educational and spiritual tours, assemblies and forums, international food aid and development, and publishing. For membership information and a current issue of the *One Peaceful World* Newsletter, including current cancer case history reports, contact: One Peaceful World, Box 10, Becket, MA 01223 (413) 623-2322.

Kushi Institute

The Kushi Institute of the Berkshires offers ongoing classes and seminars in macrobiotic cooking, health care, diagnosis, shiatsu and body energy deveopment, and philosophy. Programs include the Macrobiotic Way of Life Seminar, a two-day introductory program presented monthly; the Macrobiotic Residential Seminar, a one-week live-in program that includes hands-on training in macrobiotic cooking and home care, lectures on the philosophy and practice of macrobiotics, and meals prepared by a specially trained cooking staff; the Leadership Training Program, which offers four- and five-week intensives for individuals who wish to become trained and certified macrobiotic teachers. Similar leadership training programs are offered at Kushi Institute affiliates in Europe, and through Kushi Institute Extensions in Cleveland, Dallas, Philadelphia, New York, and other cities in North America.

The Kushi Institute also offers a variety of special programs including an annual Summer Conference in New England, special residential seminars with Michio Kushi, including Spiritual Training and Development Seminars, New Medicine Seminars, and Studies in Destiny. For information, contact: Kushi Institute of the Berkshires, Box 7, Becket MA, 01223 (413) 623-5741.

Recommended Reading

Books and publications with information on macrobiotics are available from One Peaceful World and the Kushi Institute or at other macrobiotic centers, natural foodstores, and bookstores. Ongoing developments are reported in the *One Peaceful World* Newsletter and books published by One Peaceful World Press. Moreover, Michio and Aveline Kushi and their associates have authored numerous books on macrobiotic philosophy, cooking, diet, and way of life. The following titles are especially recommended for further study:

Books by Michio Kushi

Health and Diet

1. *The Cancer-Prevention Diet* (with Alex Jack, St. Martin's Press, 1983).

2. *Diet for a Strong Heart* (with Alex Jack, St. Martin's Press, 1985).

3. *Natural Healing through Macrobiotics* (edited by Edward Esko and Marc Van Cauwenberghe, M.D., Japan Publications, 1979).

4. *Macrobiotic Home Remedies* (edited by Marc Van Cauwenberghe, M.D., Japan Publications, 1985).

5. *Macrobiotic Diet* (co-authored with Aveline Kushi; edited by Alex Jack, Japan Publications, 1985).

6. *Cancer and Heart Disease: The Macrobiotic Approach* (with various contributors; edited by Edward Esko, Japan Publications, 1986).

7. *Crime and Diet: The Macrobiotic Approach* (with various contributors; edited by Edward Esko, Japan Publications, 1987).

8. *AIDS, Macrobiotics, and Natural Immunity* (co-authored with Martha Cottrell, M.D., Japan Publications, 1990).

9. *Macrobiotic Health Education Series — Diabetes and Hypogylcemia; Allergies; Obesity, Weight Loss and Eating Disorders; Infertility and Reproductive Disorders; Arthritis; Stress and Hypertension* (with various editors, Japan Publications, 1985-88).

10. *How to See Your Health: The Book of Oriental Diagnosis* (Japan Publications, 1980)

11. *Your Face Never Lies* (Avery Publishing Group, 1983).

12. *The Macrobiotic Approach to Cancer* (with Edward Esko, Avery Publishing Group, revised edition, 1991).

Philosophy and Way of Life

1. *One Peaceful World* (with Alex Jack, St. Martin's Press, 1986).

2. *The Book of Macrobiotics: The Universal Way of Health, Happiness, and Peace* (with Alex Jack, Japan Publications, revised edition, 1986).

3. *The Macrobiotic Way* (with Stephen Blauer, Avery Publishing Group, 1985).

4. *The Book of Do-In* (Japan Publications, 1979).

5. *Macrobiotic Palm Healing: Energy at Your Fingertips* (with Olivia Oredson Saunders, Japan Publications, 1988).

6. *On the Greater View* (Avery Publishing Group, 1986).

7. *Food Governs Your Destiny* (with Aveline Kushi and Alex Jack, Japan Publications, 1986).

8. *The Gentle Art of Making Love* (with Edward and Wendy Esko, Avery Publishing Group, 1990).

9. *Other Dimensions: Exploring the Unexplained* (with Edward Esko, Avery Publishing Group, 1991).

10. *Nine Star Ki* (with Edward Esko, One Peaceful World Press, 1991).

11. *The Gospel of Peace: Jesus's Teachings of Eternal Truth* (with Alex Jack, Japan Publications, forthcoming).

Books by Aveline Kushi

Cooking

1. *Aveline Kushi's Complete Guide to Macrobiotic Cooking for Health, Harmony, and Peace* (with Alex Jack, Warner Books, 1985).

2. *Aveline Kushi's Introducing Macrobiotic Cooking* (with Wendy Esko, Japan Publications, 1987).

3. *The Changing Seasons Macrobiotic Cookbook* (with Wendy Esko, Avery Publishing Group, 1985).

4. *How to Cook with Miso* (Japan Publications, 1979).

5. *Macrobiotic Family Favorites* (with Wendy Esko, Japan Publications, 1987).

6. *The Macrobiotic Cancer Prevention Cookbook* (with Wendy Esko, Avery Publishing Group, 1988).

7. *Macrobiotic Food and Cooking Series — Diabetes and Hypoglycemia; Allergies; Obesity, Weight Loss and Eating Disorders; Infertility and Reproductive Disorders; Arthritis; Stress and Hypertension* (with various editors, Japan Publications, 1985-88).

8. *Aveline Kushi's Wonderful World of Salads* (with Wendy

Esko, Japan Publications, 1989).

9. *The Quick and Natural Macrobiotic Cookbook* (with Wendy Esko, Contemporary Books, 1989).

10. *The Good Morning Macrobiotic Breakfast Book* (with Wendy Esko, Avery Publishing Group, 1991).

11. *The New Pasta Cuisine: Low-Fat Noodle and Pasta Dishes From Around the World* (with Wendy Esko, Japan Publications, 1991).

Family Health

1. *Macrobiotic Pregnancy and Care of the Newborn* (with Michio Kushi; edited by Edward and Wendy Esko, Japan Publications, 1984).

2. *Macrobiotic Child Care and Family Health* (with Michio Kushi; edited by Edward and Wendy Esko, Japan Publications, 1986).

3. *Lessons of Night and Day* (Avery Publishing Group, 1985).

Philosophy and Way of Life

1. *Aveline: The Life and Dream of the Woman Behind Macrobiotics Today* (with Alex Jack, Japan Publications, 1988).

2. *Diet for Natural Beauty* (with Wendy Esko and Maya Tiwari, Japan Publications, 1991).

3. *Thirty Days* (with Tom Monte, Japan Publications, 1991).

Other Authors

Aihara, Herman. *Basic* Macrobiotics (Japan Publications, 1985).

Benedict, Dirk. *Confessions of a Kamikaze Cowboy* (Avery Publishing Group, 1991).

Brown, Virginia, with Susan Stayman. *Macrobiotic Miracle: How a Vermont Family Overcame Cancer* (Japan Publications, 1985).

Dietary Goals for the United States. Select Committee on Nutrition and Human Needs, U.S. Senate, 1977.

Diet, Nutrition and Cancer, National Academy of Sciences,

1982.

Dufty, William. *Sugar Blues* (Warner Books, 1975).

Esko, Edward and Wendy. *Macrobiotic Cooking for Everyone* (Japan Publications, 1980).

Esko, Edward, editor. *Doctors Look at Macrobiotics* (Japan Publications, 1988).

Heidenry, Carolyn. *Making the Transition to a Macrobiotic Diet.* (Avery Publishing Group, 1987).

Ineson, John. *The Way of Life: Macrobiotics and the Spirit of Christianity* (Japan Publications, 1986).

Jack, Alex. *Let Food Be Thy Medicine* (One Peaceful World Press, 1991).

Jack, Alex, editor, *The New Age Dictionary* (Japan Publications, 1990).

Jack, Alex and Gale. *Promenade Home: Macrobiotics and Women's Health* (Japan Publications, 1988).

Kohler, Jean and Mary Alice. *Healing Miracles from Macrobiotics* (Parker, 1979).

Nussbaum, Elaine. *Recovery: From Cancer to Health through Macrobiotics* (Japan Publications, 1986.)

Nutrition and Mental Health. Select Committee on Nutrition and Human Needs, U.S. Senate, 1977, 1980.

Ohsawa, Lima. Macrobiotic Cuisine. (Japan Publications,, 1984).

Sattilaro, Anthony, M.D., with Tom Monte. *Recalled by Life: The Story of My Recovery from Cancer* (Houghton-Mifflin, 1982).

Sergel, David. *The Macrobiotic Way of Zen Shiatsu* (Japan Publications, 1988).

Tara, William. *Macrobiotics and Human Behavior* (Japan Publications, 1985).

Yamamoto, Shizuko. *Barefoot Shiatsu* (Japan Publications, 1979).

Periodicals

One Peaceful World, Becket, Massachusetts
Macro News, Philadelphia, Pennsylvania
Macrobiotics Today, Oroville, California

About the Authors

Ann Fawcett is a writer, teacher, and counselor with a holistic and spiritual orientation. She has served as a Contributing Editor to *East West Journal* and worked at the University of Massachusetts in Amherst. She lives in Colrain, Massachusetts.

Cynthia Smith is a journalist and graduate of the Kushi Institute. She lives in Newton, Massachusetts.

About the Contributors

Norman Arnold and his wife, Gerry Sue, live in Columbia, South Carolina.

Jean Bailey lives with her family in Ontario, Canada.

Emily Bellew and her husband live in Zanesville, Ohio.

Doug Blampied is an insurance executive with Chubb Life. He lives with his wife, Nancy, in Bow, New Hampshire.

Brian Bonaventura lives in Gahanna, Ohio. He recently completed Kushi Institute Level I studies in Cleveland.

Virginia Brown, R. N., currently lives in Reading, Massachusetts. She is the the author (with Susan Stayman) of *Macrobiotic Miracle: How a Vermont Family Overcame Cancer* (Japan Publications, 1985).

Phyllis Crabtree lives in State College, Pennsylvania, with her husband, Allen.

Magdeline Cronley gives macrobiotic cooking classes in Montauk, New York.

Milenka Dobic, her husband, Bosko, and two children are actively spreading macrobiotics in their native Yugoslavia and abroad.

Cecil Dudley, now eighty-six, lives in Columbus, Ohio, where he and his wife are active in the macrobiotic community.

Hugh Faulkner, M.D., a retired General Practitioner from England, lives near Florence, Italy, with his wife, Marian.

Bill Garnell and his wife, Natalie, live in Florham Park, New Jersey, and are active in the macrobiotic community on the East Coast.

Edmund Hanley is active in the macrobiotic community in Muskegon, Michigan.

Diane Silver Hassel and her husband, a physician, teach macrobiotics in the Toronto area.

Kit Kitatani recently returned with his wife from Burma and is a senior population expert at the United Nations. He lives in the New York area with his wife and sons.

Anne Kramer lives in Washington, Michigan. She recently completed Kushi Institute Level I studies in Cleveland.

Bonnie Kramer gives macrobiotic cooking classes in Torrington, Connecticut. She is also cooking at the Kushi Institute of the Berkshires in Becket, Massachusetts.

Barbara Lee and her husband, **J. R. Lee,** are active in the macrobiotic community in Dallas. She recently completed Kushi Institute Level I studies in Dallas.

Marlene McKenna lives with her husband and child in Providence, Rhode Island, where she is a stockbroker.

Betty Metzger lives with her husband and family in Shelby, Ohio. She is involved with the macrobiotic community in Columbus.

Elaine Nussbaum is a nutritionist, teacher, and author of *Recovery* (Japan Publications, 1986). She and her family reside in West Orange, New Jersey.

Christina Pirello and her husband, Robert, are organizers of the Kushi Institute Extension Program in Philadelphia and founders of *Macro News*.

Mona Sanders and her family reside in Columbus, Mississippi.

Michael Shanik and his wife, Mickey, are presently living in Sarasota, Florida.

Bill Templeton lives in Stockbridge, Massachusetts, and teaches occasionally at the Kushi Institute of the Berkshires in Becket, Massachusetts.

Herb Walley and his wife, Virginia, run a macrobiotic bed and breakfast in Newton, Massachusetts.

Osbon Woodford is organizing macrobiotic activities in Columbus, Ohio. He recently completed Kushi Institute Level I studies in Cleveland.